HEALTHY LIVING

A Holistic Guide to *Cleansing, Revitalization* and *Nutrition*

Susana Lombardi

Founder of *We Care Holistic Health Center*

VITAL HEALTH PUBLISHING

Ridgefield, CT

Healthy Living: A Holistic Guide to *Cleansing, Revitalization* and *Nutrition*

Second edition, published in 2002 by Vital Health Publishing

First Edition Copyright © Susanna Lombardi 1997
Second Edition Copyright © Susanna Lombardi 2002

Book Design: interior, Cathy Lombardi; cover, David Richard

Published by: Vital Health Publishing
P.O. Box 152
Ridgefield, CT 06877
Website: www.vitalhealth.net
E-mail: vitalhealth@compuserve.com

Author Info: We Care Holistic Health Center
18000 Long Canyon Rd.
Desert Hot Springs, CA 92241
(760) 251-2261
(800) 888-2523

Printed in the United States of America
ISBN: 1-890612-30-8

Contents

Introduction   4

PART I   Cleansing, Revitalization, and Nutrition   6
   1   The Five Principles of Balanced Health   7
   2   Colon Detoxification   20
   3   Fasting   23
   4   Maintenance Program   29
   5   Enzymes, Your Fountain of Youth   33
   6   Easy Changes for a Healthier Life   35

PART II Food Preparation and Recipes   46
   1   Get Organized!   47
   2   Grains, Cereals, and Legumes   49
   3   Healthful Drinks   53
   4   Dressings   57
   5   Salads   61
   6   Soups   69
   7   Main Dishes   73
   8   Healthful Sweets   89
   9   Herbs   94
   10 Home Remedies   100
   11 We Care Health Center   106
   12 Testimonials   108
   Recipe Index   112

Introduction

Why This Book?

I have had extensive exposure to many aspects of the health field and have often been asked to compile a summary guide to healthful living for the participants of the We Care Revitalization Program.

The intention of this concise book is to present basic principles of good eating and self health care, providing a comprehensive survey helpful to the newcomer and of interest also to those with good previous nutritional background.

This handbook is the product of years of dedicated study of many holistic health educators and practitioners. (Through their efforts, I have synthesized the materials in this handbook.) My own varied background in the health field, as a Hatha Yoga instructor, certified lymphologist, holistic practitioner, massage, colon therapist, and director and founder of We Care, has enabled me to include a number of tips and techniques not ordinarily found in nutritional sources.

The program described herein will seldom conflict with any other therapy or treatment; however, if you are under a doctor's care, it is best to discuss this program and seek his or her counsel and support. Our program is not intended to supplant qualified health care. Not everyone needs this program, and we are not recommending it as a panacea. But there are many who will benefit from it. Note: If you suffer from a bleeding bowel or any severe bowel disturbance, it is imperative that a doctor's supervision be employed.

—Susana Lombardi

"The doctor of the future will give no medicine
but will interest his patient in the care of the human frame,
in diet and in the cause and prevention of disease."

—Thomas A. Edison

To the Reader:

The information in this book shall not be interpreted or represented as a claim for cure, diagnosis, treatment, or prevention of any disease or condition. It should be used only as educational information about utilizing nature's way of living. The concepts included in here have been practiced by thousands of people throughout the world as an alternative way of looking at the life process. Do not embark on any health regimen without consultation and approval by your doctor or health practitioner.

PART I

Cleansing
Revitalization
and
Nutrition

**The more you cleanse,
the less cravings you will have
and the easier it will be
to stay on a more healthful diet.**

1 The Five Principles of Balanced Health

The Five Principles of Balanced Health

by Dr. Mick Hall

- Detoxification and balance
- Nutrition
- Digestion
- Exercise
- Focused attention

The Facts

The U.S. Public Health Service has reported the rate of health deterioration of the American people. Out of 100 participating nations of the world, America was the healthiest in 1900. By 1920, we had dropped to the second healthiest nation. During World War II, we went back to number one—that's when sugar and meat were hard to get and family vegetable gardens were common. By 1978, we had dropped to 79th. In 1980, we were 95th! We have now hit rock bottom—that's number 100 on the list. Yet we are said to be the wealthiest nation in the world. Who or what is responsible?

A Departure from Nature

Since 1900, the basic sensible theories of health care that prevailed then have changed dramatically. The major change was the shift from nature, or natural healing methods, to drugs. This shift was accompanied by the increasing use of preservatives and chemicals and our bodies' exposure to them in food, polluted air, and synthetic fabrics. This unnatural approach to life has had a detrimental effect on the American people.

In my opinion, as long as our approach to healing (except in rare cases) involves the use of drugs, chemicals, radiation, and scalpels, we will never be truly well. If we sincerely want to restore the American people to health, or if we personally wish to reclaim our own individual health, we must return to God and follow his ways—Nature's ways—by using herbs and other natural methods that purify and strengthen the body.

The Fountain of Youth

We all look for a simple, mystical, magical something that could give the lucky discoverer a body that would no longer know the discomfort of illness or the infirmities of old age.

In one form or another, a fountain of youth has been sought by every civilization, among every generation throughout recorded history. Can you imagine a pearl of such great worth? To have a body that would stabilize at the point of maturity and never succumb to the commonly accepted course of degeneration that we refer to as disease and the aging process. The lofty dream of so many down through the ages has been to discover these magical waters. Or maybe it was a food item: a vitamin, a mineral, a drug, or some secret substance that would finally make this dream come true.

Over the past decade, our hopes have dimmed. Our enthusiastic anticipation of such a dream come true has been all but destroyed as we have observed the most advanced medical technology in history assume near total authority over our health, while at the same time failing to reduce the power that disease has over us.

We witness the death of our children from diseases that only ten years ago would have been called diseases of old age. And what hope are we given when our doctors are dying of the same degenerative diseases that are destroying millions of people right now in our own country?

Being thus preoccupied with mere survival—with arresting the process of degeneration going on inside every one of us and doing whatever we can to avoid the development of a degenerative disease—how can we sustain the hope of not only ending the disease nightmare, but stopping the aging process as well?

Obviously, if I didn't feel very confident that I have a logical solution to share with you, I would never want to focus your attention so powerfully on the dreary realities of our present health status in the U.S. I still do not believe that anyone will ever come up with any one substance to stop the process of degeneration and aging. The Five Principles of Balanced Health will clarify why this is so unlikely. But they will also show that you can stop both processes by following them.

Yes, I do believe that within the Five Principles of Balanced Health lies the secret to ageless, disease-free, balanced, and vibrant good health. Before we deal with the five principles, however, I would like to shed some light on the way degeneration takes place.

The Process of Degeneration

There is only one reason (besides pleasure) why we eat food, and that is to provide the building blocks to replace the body cells that are being destroyed as the result of what we call aging or degenerative disease. Both terms are synonymous and describe the same process. Each gives a different perspective on the same condition; premature cell destruction in the body. The body's nutritional requirements will always equal the level of cell destruction occurring in the body. This is of the utmost importance, because our primary target is to stop the cell destruction going on inside the body. If there is no cell destruction, there is no aging, thus no degeneration going on in the body. That is logical enough, isn't it?

Centuries ago human beings survived, for the most part, by eating meat. It was found that cooking it improved the flavor. As time passed, the cooking of most foods became not only a way of life but also, for many, a great art. Today, nearly all of our food is cooked before it is eaten. Although the popular trend is now toward eating more raw foods, the destruction that has taken place in the cooking process is now equaled (and replaced) by mineral and enzyme-deficient vegetables.

Let's review the process of degeneration.

At best, raw foods contain from 5 percent to 75 percent of the enzymes needed for the process of digestion. Any form of processing, such as cooking, reduces these enzyme levels drastically.

This probably doesn't seem like a real threat, since it is widely believed that "our body is meant to digest the food, the food isn't supposed to digest itself."

Raw food contains live enzymes that are meant to assist the body in the process of digestion. When our food doesn't contain these enzymes, it becomes necessary for the body to sacrifice its metabolic enzymes (the life force of the body) for the process of digestion. This sacrificing of metabolic enzymes is the fundamental physical cause of the aging process and of the process of degeneration.

A second problem, closely related to the sacrificing of metabolic enzymes, is the habit of consuming larger quantities of food than the body is capable of digesting and assimilating. These two practices—cooking and overeating—together cause a toxic buildup of undigested food residues in the colon. The result of this toxic buildup in the colon is the production of harmful bacteria, fungal overgrowth, and loss of vitality as the body struggles to neutralize the harmful element in the bowel.

While the undigested food residues are putrefying in the colon, several other systems of the body are being bogged down by an excess of waste materials: The arteries of the body are being clogged as a result of poor fat digestion. This happens when fats and oils are overheated, destroying the natural lipase enzymes and essential fatty acids. Then, with a system deficient in lecithin, the body cannot properly utilize cholesterol or fats. If the body cannot then dispose of this unusable solid fuel, it will build up and clog the arteries, restricting the circulation, which is our fueling system. This all contributes to the development of heart disease, stroke and all circulatory disorders.

Because of poor digestion, nutritional deficiencies develop throughout the body, as does metabolic imbalance. Because far more food is being put into the body than it can handle, and because there is more toxic waste in the body than all the organs of elimination are able to dispose of, tissue cells are constantly being destroyed at a very rapid pace. When we add to all of this the blocking up of the skin and the backing up of the lymphatic system, the common diagnosis of this dread disease is called "the average American adult body," tragically and unnecessarily afflicted by the aging process and the process of degeneration.

Having identified the problem, we can now proceed with the solution to the problem by discussing the Five Principles of Balanced Health.

First Principle—Detoxification and Balance

We have five organs of elimination to keep the body disease-free and operating at maximum efficiency: the colon, the skin, the lungs, the liver, and the kidneys. We also have two complete systems that play key roles in the detoxification of the body. These are the circulatory and the lymphatic systems. With so many avenues for the elimination of bodily waste, it seems we should be able to keep ahead of the accumulations that poison our cells. Unfortunately though, so many environmental conditions and misguided practices undermine our health and these organs and systems cannot keep up. Therefore, we now have a choice: Pay the consequences, or learn the Five Principles of Balanced Health and live by them.

Colon. To begin the process of detoxification, we need to start with the colon. The colon is literally the trash can of the body. If we do not empty the trash can from the kitchen for a few days, the bacterial activity in the garbage produces an offensive odor, and unwelcome insects are drawn to the smorgasbord to dine. A similar condition is found in at least 90 percent of the colons in America. I am not implying that most people do not have a bowel movement every day. I mean that today's elimination isn't always yesterday's waste. It may be from at least the day before yesterday. Any tube or pipe that constantly carries decomposition (food and body waste), accumulates a buildup on the walls. It has been found that the buildup begins shortly after the child begins to consume cooked foods, and that it continues to accumulate.

It is also estimated that 90 percent of the U.S. population has parasites. And given that almost every colon provides the perfect environment for parasitic life, this estimate is probably a conservative figure.

There are two solutions to this problem: The first is to clear the colon wall completely of the accumulated waste buildup, and the second is to balance the flora within the colon. For the best methods of properly cleansing the colon, refer to "Colon Detoxification" in the instructions section. The balancing of the intestinal flora will be dealt with in the next section—"Balance."

Skin. The next important area is detoxification of the skin. The skin is the largest organ of elimination. Second to the bowel, the skin eliminates more waste than any other organ. Because a sedentary lifestyle is so common, most people lose the tremendous benefit of the large volume of waste that could be eliminated through the skin. When the skin fails to handle its own workload, the burden must be shared by the other organs of elimination.

Of course, the most natural methods of stimulating the skin are through physical labor, exercise, and active recreation. There are also a few methods, such as dry skin brushing, scrubbing showers, herbal glow treatments, and cleansing baths, to help the body eliminate the accumulations present. It would be beneficial to follow the instructions for the cleansing bath most appropriate for your needs. Find these instructions in the section "Detoxifying Baths."

Lungs. The next organ of elimination that needs special attention is the lungs. Besides eliminating large amounts of carbon dioxide, the lungs supply us with a generous amount of oxygen. It is important to our health to keep the lungs clean and able to exchange as large a volume of air as possible. Consider the difference between a wood stove with the draft open wide, allowing a large volume of oxygen into the firebox, and thus creating a powerful, hot fire, and a similar stove with the draft nearly closed. The fire barely maintains a flame. Oxygen is just as vital to our energy production. As with any part of the body, lung capacity decreases with lack of proper use. The lungs cannot perform to the best of their ability when day after day we breathe shallowly and hardly expel all of the old air. Besides deep-breathing exercises, sports, and general aerobic exercises, the following method of detoxifying the lymphatic system is also of great benefit to the respiratory system.

Lymphatic System. Detoxifying the lymphatic system is important to the health of tissue cells as well as to all-around body hygiene. The work of the lymphatic system is to carry the blood proteins and cell waste away from tissue cells to prevent the cells from being poisoned in their own waste. When we aren't active enough, the lymphatic system slows down and doesn't properly clear the tissue of this waste. A sluggish lymphatic system allows toxic fluids to remain in the body longer than is necessary. This causes these fluids to become more toxic, and the body to dissipate its vital energy in order to protect itself from these toxic substances. A sluggish lymphatic system also restricts cell function by limiting the effectiveness of oxygen. There are two effective ways to detoxify the lymphatic system. One is the ginger bath, (instructions are in the section "Detoxifying Baths"). The second is the lymphatic exercise of bouncing on a small, round trampoline.

Balance. There are three important areas in creating balance. These are pH, bacteria, and minerals. There is perhaps no area more important, nor one that should be given a higher priority, than balancing the pH of body fluids. To maintain a constant blood pH as close to 7.4 as possible is vital to our survival. To accomplish this, the kidneys must vary the pH of the urine to compensate for diet and products of metabolism.

If a person with arthritis has an alkaline pH and is not able to balance this pH, there will always be calcium deficiencies at the same time as accumulations of excess calcium in the joint. The reason for this is that without sufficient acid, the body isn't able to hold calcium in solution.

I have yet to meet a person with cancer who can digest protein properly. Again, because of an unbalanced pH, in such a condition, the body is starving for protein and, at the same time, it is being poisoned by an excess of undigested proteins. This takes place because people who are not digesting protein, are not providing the body with sufficient hydrogen. Hydrogen (pH) acts to keep the blood pH as close to 7.4 as possible to maintain life. In the digestive process, if there is only a little more hydrogen than needed to maintain the proper pH, there isn't enough left to produce the amount of hydrochloric acid for proper digestion; therefore, the result is again poor protein digestion. Because this process could continue until death if not properly assisted, it becomes imperative to supplement the digestion to break the cycle. The use of concentrated plant enzymes accomplishes the work of digestion without excess effort on the part of the body.

The next area that must be balanced is the bacteria or intestinal flora of the colon. This balancing is just as important as the cleansing of the colon wall. There are literally hundreds of different types of bacteria in the bowel. Some are friendly bacteria, and some are destructive to our health. The balance that should be maintained is approximately 85 percent friendly bacteria to 15 percent of the Coliform or harmful bacteria. Unfortunately, in most cases, this balance is close to being just the opposite. The reason this condition is so serious is that in this state, the colon becomes a generator of harmful, disease-producing bacteria and fungal overgrowth that are hospitable to the development of more serious disease conditions.

Dr. Paul Gyorgy (discoverer of vitamin B_6) has determined that the main component of the normal human intestinal flora is lactobacillus bifidus. This bacterium establishes itself in the colon of newborns when they are fed mother's milk; it is found in the nipples of lactating mothers. This is why the use of bifidus in the rebalancing process is so important. Two effective methods of rebalancing this bacterium involve the oral use of acidophilus bifidus and rectal implants. You will find the instructions for this rebalancing in the section of instructions under "Rectal Implant."

The body also needs to be balanced in terms of minerals. This is the third area of balance, and if minerals are not in the proper balance, radiant health is an elusive dream. Space limitation makes it impossible to do justice here to the subject of minerals.

Suffice it to say that a daily intake of Power Green, whey, and chelated minerals will provide a good daily balance of minerals. Also, eliminating sugar from the diet will reduce the loss of calcium. For more on these recommendations, read the "Suggested Outline of the Average Day."

Second Principle—Nutrition

It's not what is ingested that benefits the body, but what is *digested* and *assimilated* that counts.

Nutrition is such a controversial subject. Most people who become interested in this subject soon find that they are instilled with two silent fears: The fear to eat and the fear not to eat; what supplements to take and what not to take. By the time it gets to quantities, it becomes a real concern. My own research suggests that nutrition is just as much a cause of health problems as it is a solution. There seem to be three major types of problems. The first, and most common, is *over-supplementing*. Nutritional supplements and herbal combinations have become a big business, but the average person needs guidance in establishing a reasonable program of supplementation. It is wonderful that we have the freedom to care for our individual needs as we see fit. Even so, we need to realize how concentrated these supplemental tablets and capsules are. The average health program recommends at least three times more supplementation than the body can assimilate. The body is then incapable of eliminating the supplements quickly enough, which further toxifies the body. Also, we should be concerned with the quality of those supplement products.

The second problem is the following of *special diets* that have been geared to accomplish a particular job or bring about a certain metabolic change in the system. In most cases, the target is the elimination of some type of bodily condition. Whatever the end result desired, the simple need of the body to replace destroyed tissue cells is almost always overlooked.

The third area of concern is *personal eating habits*. The one common denominator among centenarians is the eating of small quantities of food. Everything we eat has one of two fates: it must either be digested and nourish our bodies, or it must be eliminated as a waste product in a process that robs us of energy. This is why we need to consider the quality of everything we eat. If it doesn't contain the elements we want to build our body with, it should be passed over or taken in very small quantities.

I would like to share the results of an experiment to illustrate the seriousness of what I am pointing out here. Scientists took two similar groups of dogs for this experiment. To one group, they gave only water. To the other they gave water and white bread. After 30 days the group on the water was still strong and healthy. All of the group that was given water and white bread died within two weeks. Do we conclude from this that white bread is poisonous? Of course not. But again, everything that is eaten needs to be of a high enough quality to be digested and become blood, or it must be eliminated as a waste product and thereby rob the body of vital energy. So what happened to the dogs? They became fatigued to death. Through the same process, the average American is constantly half-fatigued to death at all times. But what about a little excess as long as it is good, wholesome raw food? Does it really matter what the substance is? Some foods are easier to eliminate than others and some are less toxic than others; however, food is still the building block of the body, and if the supply is in excess of the demand, the excess must be eliminated as waste. This process of eliminating the excess saps the body's vitality no matter what the food.

There are a few guidelines that I feel are important to keep in mind as you establish the nutritional program best suited to your personal needs. First of all, just as we have a spiritual belief system, and a mental belief system, I believe that the body has its own belief system. Because of our family eating habits, our bodies were built of the elements derived from a certain pattern of eating. This pattern of eating habits established a level of expectation within the body. As with any animal in nature, it is disturbing to pull the body abruptly from its comfort zone by changing the pattern of eating too rapidly. Changes in diet should be made slowly. The quickest changes should be made by eliminating from the diet as many harmful substances as possible. The body can handle doing without food completely much easier than it can adapt to drastic changes.

Conduct a careful analysis of your personal diet. Then, if the following items are a part of your daily regime, cut back and eventually eliminate them: canned meats, pork products, processed meats, processed cheese, heated oils, white sugar, white wheat flour, white rice, processed foods, fast foods, microwave meals, and canned vegetables.

Next, because the body goes through a natural cleansing cycle every day from approximately 4:00 A.M. to noon, it conflicts with nature to force the body into a feeding cycle right in the middle of a cleansing cycle. Therefore, if you are a determined breakfast person, try to satisfy your needs with fruit and a pint of lemonade until at least 11:00 A.M. before eating breakfast. The section "Average Day's Diet" will provide a clearer picture of what an average day should be like while you are following this program. (In the instruction section, please read about lemonade, so that you can understand its importance.)

The next, crucial step in the structuring of a nutrition program is to include more raw fruits and vegetables. (Read the chapter on nutrition and recipes for more help in developing a personal nutritional program.)

Third Principle—Digestion

Of all the common health complaints, the number-one cause is poor digestion. Even when there isn't heartburn, gas, indigestion, or any other obvious sign of poor digestion, there is almost no one over 20 years old with proper digestion. If you are not employing supplemental enzymes to digest food, or if at least 20 percent of your food is cooked, you have poor digestion.

The purpose of digestive enzymes excreted by the body is to help food enzymes break the food down. Our body was never meant to do all the digesting it has to do when we eat a completely cooked meal. To produce the digestive enzymes necessary for the work of digestion, the body must give up its own life force. To understand this better, let us return for a moment to the time of birth. When a body is born, it has what is called "a metabolic enzyme pool." Just like a bank account that can be added to or withdrawn from, this enzyme pool is added to as the baby nurses at its mother's breast. If the baby isn't able to nurse, it loses this additional deposit into the enzyme pool and will suffer the consequences. This enzyme pool is the level of life force within the body and is directly inherited. If the parent's enzyme pool or life force is low, the child will inherit this low level of life force. If the parents possess a healthy level of enzymes, the child inherits the high level of life force or enzyme pool. This is the major difference between a person who is basically quite robust and another who always seem to be frail or sickly.

The level of our enzyme pool and how we conserve these reserves determines the level of our health and the length of our lives. It is very common to live life burning the candle at both ends up to the age of about 40 years. Then all of a sudden, it becomes a matter of survival to step on the brakes a little and make a few lifestyle and dietary changes. This is a result of the body sending a signal that the enzyme pool is being emptied far too rapidly, and if serious changes aren't made soon, life will no longer be possible. When this enzyme pool is empty or, in other words, when our life force is gone, we call this death. Thus we are left with two areas of concern: to determine how to conserve our enzyme pool, and to replace the enzymes that have already been used up.

To conserve the enzymes we still possess, we need to stop using them. This can be accomplished by adapting a program to stop the tissue destruction: Eat more raw fruit and vegetables. The final but most powerful step is to use the correct supplemental enzymes for our personal needs.

To replace the enzymes we have already used, we need to halt the destruction of tissue cells. As you follow the Five Principals of Balanced Health, you will experience a return to the level of health that you feel was lost. As you continue following this whole program, there is one important step designed to enhance the replacement of the enzyme pool. This is the practice of drinking a pint of lemonade each morning. (The instructions for the lemonade are in the Instructions section.) The lemon is one of the most cleansing foods, especially when picked ripe. Besides its cleansing effect on the liver, the lemon also acts as a stimulator to activate the liver—a generator that is believed to turn food and supplemental enzymes into metabolic enzymes to replace what has been consumed from the metabolic pool. So do yourself a great favor and follow this program as closely as possible. Enjoy the thrill of being one of the first ever to drink from a real fountain of youth.

Fourth Principle—Exercise

Movement is life: the more movement, the more life. The fourth principle of balanced health is exercise. There are five systems of the body that need the stimulation of exercise: the lymphatic, circulatory, respiratory, organ, and muscular systems. As far as this program is concerned, exercise is necessary to assist in the process of detoxification, to tone all body tissues, to increase oxygen intake for energy, and to stimulate circulation for proper fueling of tissues cells.

I would encourage spending 10 minutes, three times a day, working out on a small, round trampoline. This is an ideal exercise. It will help clear the lymphatic system, stimulate the circulation, strengthen the heartbeat, satisfy the needs of the respiratory system, and tone every cell in the body. The mini-trampoline, brisk walks, and daily yoga are your very best exercises.

Fifth Principle—Focused Attention

The fifth principle is my favorite and I believe the most important. James Allen wrote a beautiful book expanding on the scripture: "As a man thinketh in his heart, so is he." In this little book, Allen explains so beautifully the process in which our daily thoughts solidify into the circumstances of our lives.

When we decide on a goal we want to achieve, we plan, work, dream, and finally attain the desired goal. At the time of achieving that desired goal, we are aware of the connection between the first thought of the goal and the circumstances of the achievement.

A simplified way of looking at the same process is to realize that "we always go where we are looking." Life tends to bring about circumstances that make our thoughts manifest. Undue focus on externals, whether objects or people results in a transfer of personal power (ourselves) to the object. We are no longer in command of ourselves. So be cautious of the focus of your attention. Be sure it is where you want to go.

Stop and take careful note of your daily thoughts and words. Thoughts are things! Every thought or word that you find yourself repeating, even when you are joking, is busy creating future circumstances for you. We always go where we are looking. Where are you looking? Are you sure that is where you want to go? Are you looking down the road of joy, health, happiness, love, and purpose? Is it easier for you to list your faults or your positive qualities? Which is easier for you to list, the faults or the positive qualities of those you are closely associated with? I pose these questions just to clarify the reason why it often seems as though life could be a bit brighter.

I am hoping that in this program, instead of concentrating on health problems and treatments, you will focus your attention on joyfully getting on with your healthy, happy life.

I would like to challenge you to a daily activity that I believe will help you to focus your attention. Put one of the following titles on the top left side of a sheet of paper:

1. My favorite people. (Then list the favorite people in your life.)
2. People who inspire me. (List them.)
3. Everything I am grateful for in life.
4. Everything in life that makes me happy or that I like.
5. Things I would like to do.
6. Dreams I would like to achieve.

Work every day on completing these lists until you feel comfortable with what you have written. If you have a lot to say, a notebook may be more suitable. When the lists are complete, continue by reviewing them every morning and every evening. We always go where we are looking. Get excited and inspired by where the new focus of your attention will take you.

Detoxifying Baths

Detox bath (for general detoxification and for detoxifying radiation, chemicals, and pollutants from your body). Put one full package of "detox bath" into a bath of warm water. Lie in a tub for 20 to 30 minutes and perspire. When finished, take a warm scrubbing shower. Finish the process with a cool shower. The cooler the water, the more energy you stimulate back into the body.

Chlorine bleach bath (for metal and chemical detoxification). Pour one cup of plain chlorine bleach into a full tub of warm water. Caution: Open a window or vent the room to avoid breathing fumes. Lie in a tub of this water for 20 to 30 minutes. Take a scrubbing, soapy shower after. You may want to put lotion on your body when finished.

Instructions
Before bathing, drink a hot tea and brush the skin to open the pores.

Rectal Implant

Using a rectal syringe every night while fasting, dissolve five capsules of Acidophilus in three ounces of water. Absorb water in syringe and introduce into rectum. Squeeze syringe to keep liquid in. This should be done at bedtime while lying in bed for 15 to 20 minutes. The goal is not to evacuate the intestines but to keep it inside all night.

Ten Easy Steps to Follow for Rejuvenation and Vibrant Health

1. **Air**—Oxygen is the most important element for your body function. Do three minutes of breathing exercises three times a day.
2. **Water**—Your body is 76 percent water. The quality of the water is very important to your health. Get a water purification system! Drink one half of your body weight in ounces of liquids each day. (That is, to find how many ounces you should drink each day, divide your weight in pounds by 2.)
3. **Walking**—The most simple and beneficial exercise. Enjoy a two-mile walk every day.
4. **Stretching**—Muscles that are not used will shrink. To keep flexible and young, practice yoga daily.
5. **Lymphatic exercises**—Use a mini-trampoline; it is the best way to remove poisons from your system.
6. **Cleansing the body (internally and externally)**—Clean your system with purified water, a liquid diet, periodic fasting, colon hygiene, herbs, massage, reflexology, clay packs, saunas, skin brushing, and the like. Refrain from soaking or swimming in chlorinated water.
7. **Mental and emotional cleansing**—Learn to relax and enjoy life! Let go of fears and resentments. Meditate and pray.
8. **Nutrition**—Rejuvenate with whole, natural, live foods that are full of enzymes. Refrain from eating refined, processed, devitalized, and cooked foods.
9. **Rest**—Your body rejuvenates and purifies itself with proper rest.
10. **Faith**—Learn to trust Life! Faith in life is the only real source of happiness and health!

Lemonade

Mix three ounces of freshly squeezed lemon juice into a pint of water and sweeten to taste with Stevia or maple syrup (only if you are free of candida and hypoglycemia). You may enjoy the healthy addition of a dash of cayenne pepper. Fresh lemonade will assist your body's morning cleansing cycle.

2 Colon Detoxification

The colon is the sewage system of the body. Neglected and abused, it becomes a cesspool. The cleaner your colon is, the healthier you are going to be. Your greatest keys to health are fasting one day a week and having two bowel movements per day.

Autointoxification

The process by which the body becomes poisoned from its own waste is called autointoxification. If your colon isn't clean and functioning properly, the waste matter will not be eliminated. Instead, the toxic residue will be reabsorbed into your system and will cause numerous health problems, such as bad breath, body odor, putrid gas, digestive problems, acne, prostate problems, liver and gallbladder trouble, and chronic illness. Approximately 36 known poisons can exist in the colon, including indican, ammonia, cadaerin and histidine.

Colon problems and the subject of elimination are not the most popular topics of conversation, yet millions of people are concerned. The news media constantly inform us of current statistics and accounts of people who suffer from colon-related problems. Stop and think about the following information and how it could affect you.

Laxatives. More than 40 million Americans spent $5 million on laxatives last year. This does not include the millions of dollars spent on bulking agents such as Psyllium and Metamucil.

Cancer is the second leading cause of death in the U.S. One hundred thousand people die annually from colon cancer. According to the National Cancer Society, "Evidence in recent years suggests that most colon cancer is caused by environmental agents. Some scientists believe that a diet high in beef or low in fiber is the cause."

Colitis, Ileitis, Diverticulitis, Crohn's Disease, Irritated Bowel Syndrome (IBS). These problems affect at least 32 million people and are the leading causes of hospitalization in the U.S. IBS, the number-one digestive problem, rivals the common cold in both medical costs and work loss.

Colostomy. Thousands of people worldwide have colostomies every month, each procedure requiring the removal of a portion of the colon. The person must then eliminate through an opening in the side into an attached pouch. This pouch is emptied and cleaned several times a day. Doctors who practice preventive medicine believe this drastic surgery can be prevented by a nutritional approach.

History of Colon Hydrotherapy

Colon therapy is an ancient method of treatment and form of healing. Enemas were recorded as being used as early as 1500 B.C. in the "Ebers Papyrus," an ancient Egyptian medical document.

Enemas were more common at one time than they are today. Our grandparents and great-grandparents grew up with the use of enemas as a widely accepted procedure for reversing the onset of illness. The general public's knowledge and use of this valuable health tool have decreased greatly in the past 50 years.

Benefits of a Cleansing Program

- Dissolve and break up mucoid matter
- Rapidly expel mucoid matter from the system
- Cause no cramping
- Reduce gas in the stomach and intestines
- Kill any possible infection
- Heal any sore
- Purify the blood
- Stimulate and strengthen organs, especially the heart, liver, and eliminative organs
- Increase the secretions of the liver, pancreas, and stomach
- Strengthen, heal, and rebuild the peristaltic action as well as the entire digestive system
- Take away appetite
- Calm the nervous system and reduce possible pain
- Kill some worms
- Stop any hemorrhages

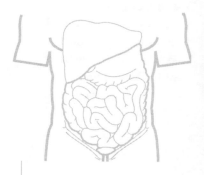

Causes of Constipation

- Too little liquid
- Too little bulk
- Too little exercise
- Emotional tension
- Mechanical problems, such as a prolapsed colon
- Poor choice of foods
- The improper combination of foods
- Very hot or cold foods
- Weak muscle tone of the colon

Constipating Foods & Drinks

- Cheese
- Fried foods
- Candies and sugar products
- White flour
- Salt and salted snack foods (potato chips, etc.)
- Beef
- Canned, burned, fermented, or processed food
- Heavy, hard-shelled, or cellulose foods, such as the tops of vegetables and legumes
- Pasteurized milk
- Wine with meals
- Carbonated drinks
- Coffee (has a drying effect on the colon)

If you are consuming these foods and drinks, your colon cannot possibly be healthy, even if you are having a bowel movement every day.

With the development of sophisticated colonic irrigation machines and the increasing desire among many people to return to more natural methods of dealing with their health, colon hydrotherapy once again is experiencing a return to popularity. It is estimated that there may be as many as 2,000 colonic therapists presently practicing in the U.S.

Colon therapists and researchers of degenerative diseases have shown that much of the body's weight can be just waste accumulated within the 60,000 miles of blood vessels, the lymphatic system, bone joints, and intra- and extracellular regions. The largest amount is found in the impactions within the colon structures: Up to 50 pounds of fecal waste can accumulate over the decades from feasting on greasy food.

Some of this partially digested, cooked food in the small intestine and colon passes into the blood stream and is deposited as waste throughout the system. If these wastes are calories, they can show up as obesity. Excess minerals show up as arthritis, excess protein is built into cancer, fat leads to high cholesterol, and sugar leads to diabetes.

Colonic irrigation, however, enables the impacted fecal matter to break down and be eliminated, along with particles of old mucus from the entire length of the colon. In some cases of cleansing, one or more forms of parasites, including tapeworms, may also be eliminated.

Colonics. A colonic is an enema given by a professional colon hygienist or therapist using a colonic machine. The procedure is quite comfortable, because the water circulates through the colon via a dual-flow tube, and no pressure is built up as a result of water retention. Colonics are usually given in a series of ten or more. In order to find a good colon hygienist, follow the recommendations of those you trust or, if possible, contact the colon hygienist society in your state.

We Care Revitalization Program

The human mechanism is an elastic pipe system. The diet of civilization is never entirely digested and the resultant waste eliminated. This entire pipe system is slowly constipated, especially at the place of the symptom and the digestive tract. This is the foundation of every disease.

To loosen this waste, eliminate it intelligently and carefully, is the goal of the We Care Revitalization Program.

3 Fasting

Fasting is a simple, quick, powerful way to cleanse the body and to help the healing process from illness and disease. Fasting one day per week, every week of your life, can become your key to a healthier life.

Fasting has been known for hundreds of years as a "compensation" against every disease. But why did it never come into general use? Because it was never used systematically, taking into account the condition of the patient. The average person has not the slightest idea what the necessary eliminative process is, what time it requires, how and how often the diet must be changed, or what it means to cleanse the body of the terrible quantities of waste that have accumulated during life.

Disease is an effort of the body to eliminate waste, mucus, and toxins, and this system assists nature in the most perfect and natural way. Remember: Your constitutional encumbrances throughout your entire system are the source of every disease: the greatest and most harmful source of lowered vitality, imperfect health, lack of strength and endurance, and any and all imperfect conditions. All have their source in the colon, never perfectly emptied since your birth.

Many people are afraid of fasting. They believe it is dangerous or detrimental to their well-being or fear that they will feel deprived. "To fast is to abstain from food while one possesses adequate reserves to nourish vital tissues; to starve is to abstain from food after reserves have been exhausted so that vital tissues are sacrificed." Fasting is a simple, quick, powerful way to cleanse the body and to enhance healing from illness and disease.

During fasting no food at all is taken, but liquids are given in great amounts. Those liquids can include delicious raw juices of fruits and vegetables, preferably fresh, because juices lose much of their valuable vitamins, minerals, trace elements, and enzymes within minutes of juicing. Vitamin-rich vegetable broth's can be utilized, as well as herb teas.

Some benefits of fasting:
1. During a fast the body lives on itself, burning and digesting its own tissues (after three days), starting with those that are diseased, damaged, aged, or dead.
2. The building of new, healthy cells is speeded up.
3. The capacity of lung, liver, kidneys, and skin is greatly increased, and masses of wastes and toxins are eliminated.
4. Fasting allows digestive, assimilative, and protective organs to rest.
5. Fasting exerts normalizing, stabilizing, and rejuvenative effects on vital physiological and mental functions.

Fasting can be done for one meal a day, for one day, or for many days at a time. Fasting is also beneficial as a general health measure. Many sources advise fasting regularly to keep the body clean. Fasting can be of value when beginning to desensitize the body to certain foods. You can see whether and how you overeat and assess your reliance on coffee, tea, smoking, alcohol, and certain foods such as refined sugar. Fasting may help you overcome those addictions.

Preparation for the Fast

Eight days prior to the beginning of the fast: Eat only fruit, raw and steamed vegetables, vegetable soups, fresh raw vegetable juices, some diluted fruit juices, herbal teas, olive oil, aloe vera juice, prune juice, and an herbal laxative tea daily.

Supplements:
3 oz. prune juice in morning
1 cup laxative tea nightly
2 T olive oil at bedtime
3 oz. aloe vera juice twice per day
Dry skin brushing: Five minutes first thing in the morning, then shower. Five minutes at bedtime, then shower (use a natural vegetable fiber brush only. Be sure not to use any oils or lotions on your skin).

Exercise:
Mini-trampoline exercises: Bounce on the rebounder at least 10 minutes per day.
Walk 20 minutes per day.
Take a detoxification bath each day.

Fasting
Seven-Day "Revitalization" Program

Have one of the following 12 drinks every hour or hour and a half. Use only distilled or purified water.

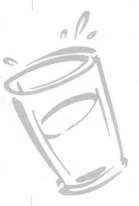

1. 2 capsules of enzymes and a glass of water
2. 3 Power Green Capsules and a glass of water
3. 1 cup of vegetable broth
4. 1st Detox—mix all ingredients, shake well, and drink fast: 8 oz. water, 2 oz. juice, 1 tsp Detox, 1 tsp Bentonite
5. 1 pint of vegetable juice (freshly made) carrot, celery, beets, cabbage
6. 2nd Detox—mix all ingredients, shake well, and drink fast: 8 oz. water, 2 oz. juice, 1 tsp Detox, 1 tsp Bentonite
7. 1 cup of lemon water (1 fresh-squeezed lemon) and 1 capsule of garlic, capsicum, and parsley
8. 1 cup of Energy Tea (1 tsp per cup of boiling water)
9. 1 cup of Blood Purifier tea (make 2 quarts and 2 T of tea, boil for 20 minutes, and refrigerate)

10. 1 cup of Liver and Kidney tea (1 tsp per cup of boiling water)
11. 3rd Detox—mix all ingredients, shake well, and drink fast: 8 oz. water, 2 oz. juice, 1 tsp Detox, 1 tsp Bentonite. Immediately followed by Whey—1 tsp in a cup of hot water. Scott's minerals—20 drops in 4 oz. of juice. Three capsules of Acidophilus (keep refrigerated).
12. 1 cup of laxative tea (1 tsp per cup of boiling water) or 3 capsules of Fiber Regulator or Aloe Vera

For best results:
- Make a rectal implant every night. (See chapter on instructions.)
- Have a shot of castor oil treatment the first day of the fast (2 oz. castor oil, mix with 4 oz. of prune or apple juice).
- Take an enema (or colema or colonic) each day.
- Jump 10 minutes on the trampoline three times a day.
- Use a sauna or steam bath each day.
- Use skin brushing twice a day.
- Walk 20 minutes and take a detoxification bath each day.
- 45 minutes of yoga stretches, breathing, and relaxation each day will help the detoxification process (yoga tape and book available).
- Repeat the Seven-Day Revitalization Program four times a year.
- Take a vacation, once or twice a year, to experience the revitalization program at We Care. We will be glad to ship all products for your home program. Call We Care at (800) 888-2523.

Breaking the Fast

The way you break your fast is very important! People have actually died breaking the fast the wrong way. I can actually tell you about a couple who were here in the year 1990. They didn't take the information seriously and on Friday, after fasting all week, they went to have fried Chinese food. Their bodies were not able to handle it, and we had to call the paramedics to pump their stomachs. So please pay attention!

The longer you fast, the longer you must be careful coming off the fast. For every week of fasting, you must be careful for two or three days.

You should not have potatoes, bananas, grains, toast, pasta, meats or cheeses. Your body may crave these foods because your body wants to stop cleansing, and these foods will do that. Watery foods are best: raw or steamed vegetables (be careful to chew your food well).

Most important, you must have small meals. You may have three, but it is better to have only two meals a day. That will also leave you time to get your drinking in. Your body needs half of its pounds of body weight in ounces of liquid a day. For example 120 lbs. = 60 oz. of liquids.

Example of small meals: a serving of steamed vegetables, a bowl of soup, a piece of fruit, or a small salad. You may add more colonics or enemas after the fast.

Remember, you have not digested any food for a week, so you must now train your body again. Say a runner is bedridden for a year. He cannot then get right up and run 20 miles. He must walk, then jog, then run.

When you leave our facility, you will want to stay on a healthy regime. We suggest the following home program and supplements in order to cleanse and rebuild your body all year long. Of course, we welcome you to return at least twice a year for our full revitalization and/or to attend one of our weekends for a mini-boost to get you back on the right track.

Coming off the fast

Instructions:
For the following three days:
- Eat very small meals.
- Eat only fresh vegetables (raw or steamed).
- Eat fresh fruit.

Breakfast
1 glass of fruit juice followed 15 minutes later by a piece of fruit

Lunch
1 glass of vegetable juice followed 15 minutes later by a vegetable salad

Dinner
1 glass of herbal tea followed 15 minutes later by a bowl of light vegetable soup

Suggested supplements

Upon rising
1 Detox drink
Fresh lemon juice in water every morning

Mid-morning
3 Power Green

With meals
Continue taking your enzymes for digestion.
Take your daily food supplement to support your nutritional needs.

At bedtime
    2 Fiber Regulator or 2 Aloe Vera capsules

Upon Completion of Cleansing, Rebuild Your Intestinal Flora
    1 box of Bifidus—3 scoops in a cup of warm water: as you get up, with your lunch, and at bedtime. Also take Acidophilus (three capsules, three times a day) for 2 weeks, then only 2 at night for maintenance.
    1 glass of kefir each morning on an empty stomach. Kefir contains beneficial bacteria and does not feed yeast. It can be made from soy or goat milk. If you make your own, at home, it has more beneficial bacteria than yogurt. Kefir has a laxative effect, it keeps the small and large intestines free from parasites. Kefir contains complete protein, many B vitamins, including B_{12}, all the essential fatty acids, and it is a natural antibiotic.

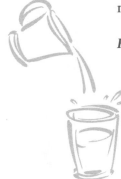

Kefir
    1 qt of milk (soy or goat)
    5 grams kefir starter culture (available at We Care)

Pour starter culture into a small glass. Pour 2 oz. of milk over the starter and stir until dissolved. Pour remaining milk into a glass container and add the dissolved mixture. Stir well. Pour all of the mixture into the kefirmaker. Plug in for 10 hrs. Then refrigerate.

Uses:
Plain, or with fruit, or over a baked potato, or on a salad.
Makes a good substitute for cream.

4 Maintenance Program

Your maintenance program should be easy to follow!

Five days per week, eat only:
fresh salads
steamed vegetables
vegetable soups
whole pastas
whole grains
legumes
seeds and nuts
fresh fruits
fresh juices and herb teas

1 day per week, fast!
1 day per week, eat anything you want!

Maintenance
Fast 1 day a week for 4 weeks.

On the fourth week (or once a month), fast for 3 days in a row (on full moon).

Every 3 months, fast for a complete week. You can do an enema in the morning and one at night.

For best results, reserve your one-week rejuvenation program at We Care twice a year.

Sample of one-day fast
Mix 1 gallon of purified water, the juice of 5 lemons, and 5 tablespoons of maple syrup or 10 drops of Stevia. Drink 1 cup every hour.

For a semi-fast
Add one simple meal a day, such as green salad, steamed vegetables, or fresh fruit.

Parasites
Parasites are the cause of many diseases. It is a healthy practice to eat foods that are natural antiparasites like pumpkin seeds, garlic, and black walnuts. Avoid foods that may have parasites like pork, sushi, or any raw or semiraw meat.

As a preventive measure, do a parasite cleanse once or twice a year with natural herbs like "Paracleanse."

Paracleanse instructions
1. Take a packet (6 capsules) in the morning and at night for 10 days.
2. Stop for 10 days.
3. Repeat the program for 10 more days.

Make sure to take lots of fluids and eat light meals (vegetables and fruits only). It can enhance your fast, but it is not necessary that you fast while taking Paracleanse.

Liver Flush (once a month, after fasting day)
Mix in blender: 4 oz. aloe vera, 2 cloves fresh garlic, 1 fresh-squeezed lemon, 3 T olive oil, 1 fresh-squeezed orange, dash of cayenne. Add 4 Liv-A (that morning).

or

On full-moon day:
Fast on juices and teas all day. Take 30 drops of Nutri-phos three times a day. At bedtime: mix 3 oz. virgin olive oil and 3 oz. lemon

juice—drink and retire immediately—next morning have an enema or a colonic

For liver weakness:

Eliminate oil or fat as much as possible, and eat absolutely no fried foods! Take 2 Liv-A twice a day, drink beet juice, eat beets (raw or steamed) in salads, have lemon juice daily, and use olive oil.

Six-Month Colon Rejuvenation Program (take daily)
- 1 glass of homemade kefir each morning
- 1 Detox in morning (1 tsp Detox, 8 oz. water, 2 oz. juice)
- 3 oz. aloe vera in a glass of juice (twice a day)
- 3 Power Green
- 2 Enzymes with each meal
- 2 Aloe Vera capsules or 2 Fiber Regulator
- 3 Acidophilus (at bedtime)

Eat lots of fibrous foods, drink lots of liquids, fast once a week, and take an enema, colema, or colonic therapy periodically.

Eighty percent of hospital admissions are for lifestyle-related preventable diseases. Some of these avoidable and reversible diseases are arteriosclerosis, coronary artery disease, arthritis, obesity, diabetes, hypoglycemia, hypertension, chronic pulmonary diseases, gastric ulcers, depression, and stress-related illness.

Daily Maintenance Supplements
Package #1
Includes the folllowing help for digestion, assimilation, and elimination:
- **Detox Drink**—Fiber to remove debris from the colon (organic ground flax seed, oat bran, apple pectin, slippery elm, psyllium)
- **Enzymes**—Break down food to help digestion (amylase to digest carbohydrates, protease for protein, lactase for lactose, lipase for fats, cellulase for cellulose)
- **Power Green Capsules**—Instant energy food (chlorophyll, chlorella, spirulina, alfalfa, barley and wheat grasses, dulse, and kelp)
- **Kyodophilus**—Reintroduces beneficial bacteria into intestine (acidophilus, bifidum, and longum)
- **Colloidal Minerals**—for daily requirement (helps absorb vitamins)
- **Fiber Regulator or Aloe Vera Capsules**—(natural laxative)

Package #2—High Performance
Reach your goal of high energy and health by using these items regularly (whole super foods dehydrated into a powder)
- **My Whey**—Proteins and minerals from goat milk (coffee replacement)
- **Yerba Mate**—Energy tea (can be used as coffee replacement)
- **Essential Light**—Complete nutrition from barley and kamut grass, rice bran, lecithin, goat whey
- **Integris**—Balances blood sugar throughout the day (Made from rice bran, it contains essential fatty acids, B vitamins, antioxidants, and CQ-10.)
- **Lecithin**—Brain food and weight-loss helper

Other:
Bio salt—Twelve tissue salts (a salt replacment)
Stevia—No calories (a sugar replacement)
My Protein—Instant energy bouillon
Vitamin C
Vitamins A and D
Calcium and Magnesium—for healthy bones
MSM—natural anti-inflammatory

5 Enzymes, Your Fountain of Youth

It is not what you eat but what you digest and assimilate that will increase your energy and vitality. Enzymes help to break down the food for proper assimilation of nutrients.

A Healthy Diet

Sixty-five percent raw foods (fresh juices, salads, nut milk, and fruit). Thirty-five percent cooked foods (steamed vegetables, grains, and legumes).

Grains

Grains are seeds that need to be soaked overnight and cooked in the same water.

Nuts and Seeds

These must be soaked overnight for the enzymes to be released. The five best nuts and seeds are almonds, sesame, pumpkin, sunflower, and apricot kernels, because they are the most balanced. Some of the others are acid-forming and constipating.

Legumes

Legumes must also be soaked overnight, but the water should be thrown away because it creates gas. Cook in fresh water.

Energy

Sixty percent of our energy is spent trying to digest food. The better you feed your body (with easy-to-digest foods), the more energy you will have. Easy-to-digest foods include liquid meals, juices, fruits, and vegetables.

Enzymes

Enzymes are a part of every living cell. There are about 100,000 enzymes in every cell. Enzymes transform grape juice into wine, barley into beer, and apple into the nutrients that your body needs. You need these enzymes to digest your foods. Once enzymes have completed their appointed task, they are destroyed. You need a constant supply of enzymes. An enzyme deficiency must be considered as a possible precursor to bodily imbalance and consequent disease symptoms. Enzymes should be supplemented in the diet just as we supplement minerals and vitamins.

The enzymes are located in the foods you eat and in your body. They are the digestive juices your body produces when it digests foods. When you eat cooked foods (foods with no enzymes), your body overworks, because it must produce twice as much digestive enzymes! Rejuvenate by fasting and eating raw foods.

Foods that contain enzymes include raw fresh vegetables and fruits, nuts and seeds (unroasted), fresh eggs (if you find a good source), and raw goat's milk.

Drink your enzymes: Your freshly squeezed raw vegetable juice has the highest content of enzymes.

The biggest enemy of enzymes is heat. In anything that has been heated up to 118 degrees, the enzymes have been totally destroyed.

To Produce Enzymatic Power to Digest Our Foods, We Must:

1. **Relax.** You need to relax and have a clear mind when you eat. If you are tense, you cannot secrete the enzymes needed to digest your food properly. We tend to do the opposite—when we've just had an argument with a lover or friend, the first thing we do is go to the refrigerator.

2. **Chew well.** The more you chew, the less work your body has to do to break down food. Foods need to be transformed into a liquid, and then into molecules that pass through the walls of the intestine into the blood stream to nourish the cells.

3. **Do not drink with your meals.** Doing so dilutes the digestive juices that break down the food. Drink 1/2 hour before your meal or 2 hours after your meal. Drink, in ounces, half of your body weight in pounds every day.

4. **Avoid hot or cold.** Don't drink your liquids too hot because they can burn the lining in your stomach (where the enzymes are produced). Drinking very cold things puts the enzymes into a dormant stage.

5. **Eat only when your stomach is empty.** Wait 4 to 5 hours between solid meals and have liquid meals in between.

6 Easy Changes for a Healthier Life

Easy does it! Do not get overwhelmed.
Just take it one step at a time.

1. Avoid packaged meats such as bologna, salami, ham, sausages, hot dogs, and turkey (compressed meats with preservatives, additives, and the like).
2. Pork and ham have the highest content of fat. These animals often carry parasites.
3. Beef also has a high content of fat, and it is in the fat that chemicals accumulate.
4. Fish contain all the poisons that we are throwing in the ocean. Industrial companies are dumping large quantities of mercury, and whole colonies of fish are dying.
5. Commercial chicken and eggs are full of hormones that are introduced for quicker reproduction and are then passed down to you. This affects your glandular system.

Suggested Reading: *Diet for a New America* by John Robbins

Flour. The center of the grain is white starch or glue, and the outside is a brown shell that contains all the oils and nutrients. The white flour or white rice is obtained by a chemical process in which the outside is shaved off, leaving just the nutrientless inside. This process exists because commercially it is more productive. If the grain were whole, it would need to be refrigerated and would spoil in a short time. By using white, refined products, producers avoid the need to use refrigerated trucks to transport them and have absolutely no product waste. Please eliminate all white flour products.

Whole Grains. Change your diet over to whole grains. Remember that the whole grains must be soaked overnight. This process will convert the center of the grain (starch) into a little leaf, which is then protein. Our bodies are not designed to digest the white flour; therefore, to be able to handle it, the body must take from its own reserve of minerals which are stored in the bones. (The bones are the storehouse of vitamins and minerals.).

Sugar. The composition of the mineral content of your blood is changed by sugar. It especially affects calcium, sodium, and potassium. Eliminate all white sugar intake. Reduce other sugars, dextrose, maltose, fructose, maple syrup, corn syrup, brown sugar, honey, etc. They all have the same effect in your body. The best sugar is rice bran syrup, molasses, and Stevia. Limit the intake of fresh fruits to one or two a day. Drink little or no fruit juices (one glass of fruit juice equals six to eight pieces of fruit).

Cooked Fats. Oil is a very important nutrient. You need no more than two tablespoons per day to lubricate the joints in the body. Good oil means raw, cold-pressed or cold-spelled. If this is not indicated on the label, it is not a good oil. Cooked oils and fats, and oils pressed under heat, change in molecular structure, becoming a solid molecule that your body cannot use for lubrication. These molecules stay in the veins and arteries, causing cholesterol buildup, hardening of the arteries, arteriosclerosis, and heart disease.

Good oils include virgin olive oil and a cold-press combination of flax and sunflower oil by Omega (Essential Balance). Other cold-press oils are avocado, almond, and sesame oil. Eliminate anything that is hydrogenated or pasteurized, such as margarine, Crisco, and the like. Do not cook with oil; cook with water and serve the oil at the table. Keep oil refrigerated, and buy it in small amounts or it will spoil.

Dairy Products. These are mucus-forming. They contain fat, many chemicals and pesticides, and they cause constipation. Use small amounts of nonpasteurized goat milk and goat cheese or soy cheese. Substitute nut milk for cow's milk; nut butter for butter; soy cheese for cheese, and occasionally use goat cheese.

Protein. We need protein in small amounts which is found in all vegetables, grains, legumes, sprouts, and seeds. Most vegetable protein is an incomplete protein, which means it does not contain all the essential amino acids. Consequently, you must learn to eat a wide variety of foods. Nutritious foods high in protein include avocado, nuts, seeds, sprouts, grains, legumes, and tofu.

If you still eat meat, fish, or chicken, eat it in small amounts and buy free-range chicken at the health store. You can mix these meats with steamed vegetables, salad, or soups. Do not mix them with bread, pasta, grain, or baked potato. The best way to cook the meat is on the broiler, letting the fat drip away.

Fruit. Eat fruit alone. Fruit is a healthful snack, and eating one to two pieces of fruit per day is desirable. You can have fruit one half hour before your meals or 2 hours after your meals.

Nutritional Program

Daily nutrition should include:
- 1 pint of fresh vegetable juice
- 1 glass of lemon water (1 freshly squeezed lemon)
- 3 Power Green capsules
- 1 large bowl of fresh, green salad, including sprouts
- 1 or 2 pieces of fruit
- 2 c of herb tea
- 1 c of goat whey or miso
- 1 c of homemade kefir from goat's milk
- 1 portion of nut milk
- Other foods to alternate: steamed vegetables, vegetable soups, grains, legumes, whole pasta, and tofu

Examples of Healthy Food Combinations:
- Grains plus nuts and seeds
- Grains and legumes
- Avocado and sprouts
- Salads sprouts and seeds
- Rice and beans with a salad
- Steamed vegetables with rice and nuts
- Baked potato, nut milk, and a salad
- Fruit and nut milk or kefir
- Soft-boiled, fertile eggs from free-range chickens could be a good source of protein during your transition diet.

Foods to Avoid

- Dairy products such as milk, cheese, butter, etc.
- Refined carbohydrates such as sugar, white flour, white rice, pastries, cake, and breads
- Tea
- Coffee
- Chocolate
- Carbonated drinks
- Alcohol
- Tap water
- Dried fruit (use very little, and soak them)
- Vinegar (use lemon instead)
- Pork, red meats, shellfish, dark poultry, rabbits, organ meats
- Roasted and salted seeds and nuts (eat only raw or nut milk)
- Fried foods
- Fruit juices (very little—diluted only)
- Canned foods
- Cold cuts such as salami, bologna, ham,
- Hot dogs

Average day's diet

Upon rising
1 glass of water
30 minutes later, herbal tea and detox drink
30 minutes later, juice of a fresh lemon in a glass of water

Breakfast
- Smoothie: nut milk or kefir and a piece of fruit in the blender (You may add 1 T of Essential Light or 1 T of My Whey, Integris, or Lecithin)
- Fresh vegetable juice (carrot, celery, beet, cabbage)

Mid-morning
Energy Tea

Lunch
1 enzyme, multiple-vitamin and mineral tablet before lunch
Fresh green vegetable salad with sprouts and nut milk
(You may add baked potato, bowl of brown rice, or slice of flourless bread.)

2 1/2 hours after lunch
Water, herb tea, and lapacho tea

Mid-afternoon
3 Power Green

Early dinner
2 enzyme tablets before dinner
Choose two or three of the following: salad, steamed vegetables, bowl of soup, noodles or grain or flourless bread, legumes and grains, avocado and sprouts (sandwich, salad), tofu or soyburgers.

Evening
1 cup of goat's whey

Bedtime
2 Acidophilus tablets every night for maintenance

My Whey, Essential Light, Kefir Starter, Stevia, My Protein, Bio-Salt, Integris, and other products are available at We Care.

Guide to Shopping
Shopping List
Buy organically grown food at your local health food stores.

Grains
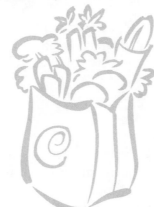

Millet
Quinoa
Brown rice
Basmati brown rice
Wild rice
Steel-cut oats
Wheat kernels
Cracked wheat
Rye
Corn
Buckwheat
Spelt
Buy whole grains, (brands like Arrowhead Mills, Harvest Quinoa, Lundburg, Now Foods, etc.) and healthful packaged hot and cold cereals and granola from organically grown, sugar and salt-free whole grains (brands like Arrowhead Mills, Healthy Valley, Bread Shop, Familia, Very Pure, Life Stream, Nature's Path).

Pasta and noodles made from:
Artichoke and semolina
Quinoa and semolina
Whole wheat
Whole durham flour
Corn
Oats
Rice
Spelt
(Brands: De Boles, El Molino, Ancient Harvest Quinoa, Annie Chun's)
Avoid white, enriched or bleached flour.

Breads, Pastries, and Crackers
Best are those made from sprouted wheat, rye, and seven grains (100 percent flourless).
Whole wheat pita bread
Blue corn tortillas
Chapaties
(Brands: Oasis, Food for Life, Essene, Garden of Eden, French Meadow, Rudolph's, Nature's Path)
Avoid white, enriched or bleached flour.

Best Oils

- Omega essential balance
- Virgin olive oil
- Flax seed oil

Oils to Avoid

Hydrogenated and transfat

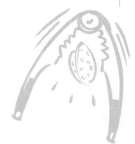

Coffee:

Highly acid-forming

Substitute:

Yerba Mate

My Whey

Grain coffee

Best Sweeteners

- Stevia
- Rice bran syrup

Oils

Total: 2 T per day (a small portion of each):

Flax seed oil (Omega's Essential Balance)

Virgin olive oil

Cold-pressed almond, avocado, sesame, sunflower, and canola

Raw butter or ghee (optional, small portion)

Nut butters

Almond butter

Sesame tahini butter

Cashew butter

Sunflower butter

Peanut butter (occasionally)

Avoid margarine, vegetable shortening, and animal fats.

Seeds and nuts for nut milk (raw and unsalted)

Almonds

Sesame seeds

Sunflower seeds

Pumpkin seeds

Cashews

Legumes

Beans: adzuki, pinto, black, kidney and mung, etc.

Lentils

Garbanzo beans

Chick peas

Fesh or frozen Edamame (soy beans)

Beverages

Soy milk

Rice milk

Almond milk

Amasake

Fresh Ferraros, Hansen juices, others—organic herbal teas

Coffee substitute, such as Herbal Beverage, Roma, and My Whey.

Herbal teas

Purified water

Sweeteners

Stevia (noncaloric, made from the chrysanthemum flower, good for diabetics and hypoglycemia)

(Brands: Now Foods, Wisdom of the Ancients)

Cinnamon powder
Rice bran syrup (fructose-free)
Occasionally:
Maple syrup
Date crystals
Barley malt syrup
Honey

Seasonings
Bio-Salt (salt substitute)
Cayenne (pepper substitute)
Kelp
Fresh and dried herbs
Fresh lemon juice
Vinegar: unfiltered and unpasteurized, apple cider
My-Protein: (noncaloric dressing; delicious for salads, soups, rice, noodles, and sauces.)
Carob: (chocolate substitute) high in calcium and fiber
Cinnamon
Nutmeg
Natural vanilla extract
Nutritional yeast: (good cheese flavor for salads and soups); full of B-complex. Do not substitute brewer's yeast—Kal brand.
Miso paste: barley and rice miso (for soups); rich in B-complex. Buy unpasteurized. Avoid boiling.
Tofu: low cholesterol and low in calories. Source of protein.
Tempeh: like tofu, low in fat and calories and rich in nutrients. Made from soybeans.
Agar-agar: tasteless, noncaloric vegetable gelatin from seaweed.
Arrowroot: (to thicken sauces and soups); replacement for cornstarch.

Sea Vegetables (Iodine and Minerals)
Dulse
Wakame
Nori

Cheeses
Soy cheese
Goat cheese (occasionally)
Tofutti from soy (better than cream cheese)
Rice cheese
Seed cheese

Best Vinegar
Organic—unpasteurized apple cider
Other vinegars are acid-forming.

Candida Diet:

Almost restricted to green leafy vegetables and grains like millet and quinoa

- No wheat
- No sugar
- No fruit juices
- Just one piece of fruit a day
- No dairy products, vinegar, soy sauce, sweets of any kind
- Increase your intake of acidophilus
- Keep cleansing the body
- No fermented foods
- No alcohol

Note:

For more information on the Candida diet, please call our office.

Further Suggestions

Condiments:
Bio-Salt, kelp, garlic, oregano, veggie salt, cayenne pepper, lemon, onion powder, basil

Juices:
Fresh vegetable (15 minutes before your meals)

Herb teas:
Yerba Mate, Lapacho, Swiss Kriss, etc.

Use:
Olive oil and lemon, My-Protein, tahini butter, almond butter, miso, and tahini dressing.
Fish and poultry: occasional use only; not recommended

Breakfast Ideas

1. Piece of fruit
2. 1 cup of kefir
3. Melons (alone)
4. Breakfast drink (mix in blender). Choose one:
   a. Orange, lemon juice, banana, apple, ground pumpkin seeds, carrot, beet
   b. Raisins, coconut, banana, papaya, water
   c. Apple, banana, orange, water, raisins, almonds
   d. Avocado, cashews, banana, coconut, water
   e. To improve nutrition and flavor, add 1 T of My Whey or 1 T of Essential Light or 1 T of Kyogreen to any of the above.
5. Whole-grain cereal (cooked) and served with nut milk. Choose one:
   a. Millet
   b. Quinoa
   c. Oat
   d. Rye
   e. Seven grain
6. Fresh fruit (then wait 20 minutes) uncooked cereal (Familia) or cooked grain
7. Poached or soft-boiled eggs, sprouted grain bread, nut butter (raw sesame tahini or almond)

Lunch or Dinner Ideas

1. Raw fruit salad (melons alone) plus goat kefir or yogurt or nut milk

2. Large vegetable salad (celery, spinach, cucumber, carrots, bell pepper, radishes, alfalfa sprouts or sunflower seeds, etc.) plus sprouted-grain bread or cracker, brown rice, ground seeds, soup, or broth

3. Homemade vegetable soup plus small salad, baked potato, crackers or sprouted-grain bread, sesame butter

4. Steamed vegetables plus sprouted-grain bread or crackers, small salad, brown rice

5. Avocado and alfalfa sandwich with sprouted-grain bread, tomatoes, miso or raw sesame tahini, and an apple

6. Fish, baked or broiled, plus cooked vegetables, small salad

7. Brown rice and beans (or any other legume) plus small salad, cup of soup, corn tortilla

8. Soup plus sprouted-grain bread, nut butter. Types of soup: vegetable, lentil, broccoli, miso broth, miso and mixed vegetable

9. Fertile eggs, goat cheeses, and fish may be eaten occasionally.

Summary

To be able to stay on a healthful diet composed of lots of fresh organic vegetables and fruits with some grains, legumes, seeds, and nuts, your body must be maintained "clean." If your body is kept clean, you will not crave meats, fried foods, sugar, and other processed foods.

The practice of a 1-day fast every week, and a 1-week cleansing every 3 months is your best tool to accomplish this.

Get your kitchen organized! Throw out all white flour, sugar, and canned food. Read labels! Do your shopping once a week, washing, drying, and packaging all your fresh vegetables and fruits. Prepare several dressings all at once to season your salads, steamed vegetables, noodles, grains, and so on. Cook extra rice, beans, lentils, and tomato sauce, and freeze an extra portion for "instant meals." Drink fresh vegetable juice and lemon juice daily! Eat lots of salads and sprouts.

Create your own support group! Invite a couple of "Health Advocate" friends to a potluck to discuss, learn, and promote healthful living.

Buy books, magazines, cassettes, and videos containing health and environmental information to share. Support organizations dedicated to health research and enlightenment. Be an example!

And, remember: Movement is life! Breathing exercises, walks, yoga, and trampoline exercise must be incorporated into your daily routine for a healthier life.

Example:

1. Fast 1 day per week (drink hourly) or semi-fast (add only one simple meal, such as:
   Green salad
   Steamed vegetables
   Vegetable soup
   Fruit plate

2. Drink lots of fluids daily (every 1 1/2 hours)
   Purified water
   Water and lemon
   Vegetable juice
   Small fruit juice
   Essential Light
   My Whey
   Kyogreen
   Power Green
   Smoothies
   Vegetable soup

3. Have two to three bowel movements daily
   Take 1 tsp of Detox daily, and drink lots of water.
   Take natural laxatives as needed. Alternate:
   Kefir
   Prune juice
   Aloe vera juice
   Fiber Regulator
   Aloe Vera capsules
   Magnesium
   Cascara sagrada
   Swiss Kriss
   Olive oil
   Castor oil

4. On full-moon day (repeat every month):
   Fast, have an enema or colonic. Do a liver flush. Fast all day, have 30 drops of Nutriphos three times a day. At bedtime, drink 3 oz. of fresh-squeezed lemon juice and 3 oz. of olive oil. Next morning, have an enema or colonic.

5. Eat lots of vegetables and fresh fruits:
   raw salads, steam, grill, sautéed vegetables, soups.

6. Eat only whole grains, legumes, seeds, and nuts.

7. Avoid nonfoods:
   cold cuts
   hot dogs
   pork meat
   dairy products

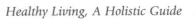

fried foods
white flour
white sugar
canned food
coffee
sodas

8. Learn to switch:
    from milk to: nut milk, soy milk, rice milk
    from cheese to: soy cheese, small amount of goat cheese
    from white-flour bread to: whole wheat, whole grains, sprouted grains
    from white pasta to: whole durham, quinoa, spelt, Jerusalem artichoke
    from oil to: virgin olive oil, Omega essential balanced oil, flax oil
    from margarine and butter to: nut butter (almond and sesame)
    from regular ketchup to: Heinz ketchup (no sugar)
    from regular mustard to: Heinz, or Westbrae mustard
    from coffee to: grain coffee, My Whey, Yerba Mate
    from white sugar to: Stevia, rice bran syrup, honey or maple syrup
    from canned foods to: fresh and frozen vegetables

9. To help digestion, eat only two solid meals. Eat early during day hours. Have 2 capsules of enzymes before meals.

10. Get organized! Shop once a week. Wash, dry, and pack every vegetable. Prepare three dressings, enough for the week. Cook enough rice, beans, soups, etc.

11. When going out to eat, choose only healthy restaurants, order à la carte, specify a dressing of lemon and olive oil.

12. Exercise daily: walks, yoga, and trampoline.

When making health changes: Do not get overwhelmed.
- Make a *few* changes at a time
- You do not have to be perfect, just *better*
- *Any* improvement is an improvement!

PART II

Food
Preparation
and
Recipes

Make food taste good to you!
Feel free to add (or remove)
any ingredient that you like
(or dislike) in any recipe.
Cooking is fun!

7 Get Organized!

Abbreviations

c—cup

T—tablespoon

t—teaspoon

oil—only virgin olive oil
or Omega's Essential
Balance

Preparation Tips

1. Eat at home and shop at health food stores for vegetables and fruits, preferably organically grown.
2. Use purified water in cooking and drinking.
3. Use stainless steel, NO aluminum cookware, NO microwave cooking, foil, or Teflon-coated cookware.
4. Do your shopping once or twice per week.
5. Soak all fruits and vegetables in a sink full of water and 1 c of lemon juice or vinegar for 15 minutes; then rinse again with water. Dry them well in spinner and store them in Ziplock bags.
6. Have a tray of salad vegetables clean and ready to go.
7. Have another tray ready to go for steamed vegetables.
8. Prepare four dressings of your choice (enough for a week). Use them freely over salads, steamed vegetables, pastas, grains, legumes, baked potatoes, and as dressing for sandwiches.
9. Add oil and Bio-Salt after the food is cooked (oil and salt should not be heated).
10. Use vegetables and fruits that are fresh, not frozen or canned (eat raw foods as much as possible). If vegetables are cooked, they should be lightly steamed or baked.

How to Steam Your Vegetables

It takes practice to be able to steam the vegetables so that they are tender but not overcooked. In general, steam the harder vegetables such as broccoli and cauliflower first, and add the softer vegetables such as mushrooms and squash toward the end.

Fill the pan with enough water (usually to the 1/2-inch to 3/4-inch level) and flush with the bottom surface of the steamer. Place the steamer inside, and cover until the water boils. Then add the vegetables, cover, and turn the heat to medium. Steam to desired texture.

Emphasize broccoli, zucchini, and string beans in your cleansing diet.

8 Grains, Cereals, and Legumes

When you are on a vegetarian diet, whole grains and legumes are your staple food. They are a great source of protein, vitamins, and minerals.

Good Sources of
Protein
Natural Fats
Complex Carbohydrate
B Vitamins
Fiber

Whole Grains:
Quinoa
Millet
Brown rice
Corn
Wheat
Oat
Rye
Buckwheat
Barley
Amaranth
Tritricale
Spelt

Whole grains are vegetarians' staple food. They contain B vitamins, minerals, complex carbohydrates, protein, and fiber. Purchase a variety of whole grains, and store them in a cool place. Soak them overnight and rinse before cooking.

Directions:
1 c of grain to 2 1/2 c of water
Corn meal (polenta) needs 4 cups of water per cup. Cooking time varies from 20 minutes to 1 hour. Bring to a boil; then reduce heat to low and cook until tender. Grains can be served for breakfast or lunch by pouring one of the following:
Do not use milk—use nut milk instead or nut butter: almond, cashew or tahini.
Or: Add olive oil and My-Protein.
Or: Add tahini dressing.
Or: Add 4 c of chopped veggies (onions, garlic, parsley, carrots, zucchini, green peas, etc.) Cook together and serve.
Or: Save leftover cooked grain to add to salads, soups, or steamed vegetables.

Nut Milk
Buy raw organic seeds and nuts (not roasted or salted). Keep them in a cool place.

Soak overnight:

2 T of each: Almonds, pumpkin, sesame, and sunflower seeds.
Add 1/2 quart of water and vanilla extract, cinnamon, or 1 date to
sweeten. Blend and serve over grains. Save leftover nut milk in
refrigerator (it is good for three days).

Or: Make a smoothie by adding a piece of fruit and a few ice cubes.
To improve nutrition and flavor, add 1 T of Essential Light or 1 T of My
Whey, Integris, or Lecithin to smoothie.

Cold Mixed Cereal
   2 c rolled oats
   1/2 c rolled wheat
   1/2 c rolled rye
   1/4 c chopped raisins
   1/4 c chopped dates
   2 T honey
   1/4 c oat bran
   1/2 c finely chopped almonds, lightly toasted
   1/2 c finely chopped sesame and sunflower seeds, lightly toasted
   1/4 c finely chopped dried apricots

*Stir together all ingredients in a mixing bowl. Transfer to a tightly covered
container. Store in a cool place. Serve with nut milk or soy milk. Allow to
soak until grains are soft.*

Quick Hot Cereal
   1 apple, grated
   1/4 c raisins
   1/2 c grated carrots
   (Use leftover pulp from carrot juice.)
   1 c of oat bran
   2 1/4 c of water

*Mix all ingredients in a pan. Bring to a boil, stirring constantly. Lower
heat and simmer 3 minutes. Remove from heat. Cover and let stand 5
minutes. (Serve nut milk over cereal.)*

Beans

All beans should be sprouted (soaked in water overnight) before cooking to discourage their tendency to cause gas. When cooking grains and legumes, add chopped vegetables to improve flavor. Cook enough grains and legumes for three or four extra meals; store foods in small containers in your freezer.

Legumes
Beans
Garbanzos
Lentils
Peas
Soybeans

Nuts and seeds:
Almonds
Sesame seeds
Sunflower seeds
Pumpkin seeds
Cashews

Grains:
Millet
Quinoa
Brown rice
Corn
Oats
Rye
Whole wheat
Barley
Spelt
Buckwheat

9 Healthful Drinks and Smoothies

At We Care, we suggest eating only:
Two solid meals and several liquid meals (every 1 1/2 hours)
every day. Lots of fresh vegetable juices. Some fresh fruit
juices. Herbal teas, lemon water, and smoothies. Following
this plan will help your nutrition and elimination. Liquid
meals are an instant source of excellent nutrition.

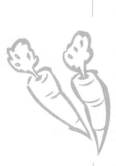

Vegetable juices

An abundance of fresh, raw juices will help the body release toxins, leaving us energized and healthy. We will begin to see an improvement in our skin and our hair. Many people who have followed the juice therapy have reported increased flexibility in arthritic joints; colds and flus disappear effortlessly; eyesight improves; and serious illnesses have often improved dramatically.

Juice #1
> 6 oz. carrot
> 1 oz. beet
> 3 oz. celery

Juice #2
> 3 oz. lettuce
> 1 oz. beet
> 2 oz. celery

Let's give our digestive system a break; let's take a rejuvenation vacation!

Let's have a fresh vegetable juice every day!

Juice #3
> 7 oz. celery
> 5 oz. lettuce
> 4 oz. spinach

Juice #4
> 6 oz. carrot
> 2 oz. apple
> 2 oz. orange
> 1 oz. lemon

Suggested Reading:

Fresh Vegetable and Fruit Juices
by Dr. N. W. Walker

Juice #5
> 6 oz. grapefruit
> 3 oz. lemon
> 7 oz. apple
> 2 oz. celery

Juice #6
> 3 oz. carrot
> 1 oz. beet
> 1 oz. lemon

Juice #7
> 1 oz. beet
> 2 oz. spinach
> 7 oz. orange

Juice #8
   6 oz. grapefruit
   3 oz. lemon

Green Nut Juice
   15 almonds soaked overnight in warm water
   4 dates pitted and soaked overnight in warm water
   5 t sunflower seeds soaked overnight in warm water
   8 oz. fresh pineapple juice

   Put in blender and mix. Set aside. Add 8 oz. more of fresh pineapple juice. Put in blender. Then fill to the top with spinach, beet tops, dandelion, watercress, and endive. Blend all together. Add 1 t bee pollen, and mix the two blends together.

Fruit drinks and smoothies

According to Dr. Ann Wigmore, 90% of our population has severe digestive problems. In her opinion, blending our food is an excellent solution. It is a fun way to make delicious after-school smoothies for the kids and for yourself!

An excellent blender/food processor is the Vita-Mix. It can help you prepare fruit and vegetable juices, vegetable soup, dressings, ice cream, sorbets, smoothies, nut butters. It also crushes ice and shreds foods instantly.

Hint:
When fruit is frozen, you get a thicker, colder, creamier smoothie.

Fruit drinks and smoothies

Create different smoothies by changing the fruit, or the fruit juices, or by adding soy milk or rice milk.
   1. Apple juice, banana, strawberries, ice
   2. Apple juice, cantaloupe, watermelon, banana, ice
   3. Banana, nut milk, soy milk, or kefir, strawberries, ice (sweeten with Stevia)
   4. Banana, mango, orange juice, ice
   5. Tropical fruit juice, raspberries, boysenberries, peaches

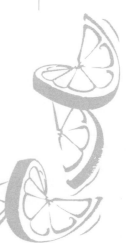

For a more nutritional drink, add one or several of the following ingredients:

   1 T of Essential Light
   1 T of Lecithin
   1 T of My Whey
   1 T of Integris
   1 T of Kyogreen
   1 T of Detox (fiber)
To improve flavor add 1/2 t of Vanilla and/or 1 T of Carob Powder.

Café Latte

> *To a cup of hot water, add:*
> 1 T of My Whey
> 1 T of Bifidus
> Dash of Carob Powder
> 1/4 t of Vanilla
>
> *Mix and drink as a coffee replacement.*

For a more decorative look, pour this mixture into a blender for a few seconds, then serve.

10 Dressings

Dressings are fun to prepare and add flavor to your food. Once a week, prepare 3 or 4 different dressings, enough to last for the whole week. The same dressing can be used over salads, steamed vegetables, brown rice, noodles, and sandwiches.

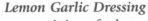

Lemon Garlic Dressing

juice of a lemon
1 clove garlic
cloves
1 yellow onion
1 t oregano
1/2 t kelp
olive oil optional

Mix in blender. Allow flavors to blend in refrigerator.

Italian Herbal Dressing

3 large tomatoes
1/2 peeled cucumber
1 yellow onion
1 clove garlic
dash of cayenne
1 t dill
2 T lemon juice
olive oil optional

Mix above ingredients in a blender. Chill to allow flavors to blend.

Avocado Green Dressing

2 t My-Protein, season to taste
1 medium avocado, ripened
juice of 1/2 lemon
1 clove garlic
1 pinch of cayenne (optional)

Mix in blender.

"Kelp from the Sea" Dressing

2-3 T lemon juice
1 clove garlic
1 yellow onion
1/2 t kelp
1/2 t My-Protein
1 t oregano

Mix in blender. Allow flavors to blend in refrigerator.

Dynamic Herbal Dressing
   2/3 c lemon juice
   3 scallions
   1/4 c parsley
   1/3 t each oregano and rosemary
   1/2 t cayenne
   1/2 t celery seed
   1/2 t basil

   Mix in blender and chill for 1 hour before serving.

Cleansing Chili Sauce
   3 tomatoes
   1 green pepper
   1/2 t oregano
   1/8 t cayenne
   1/4 c green onions
   1-2 t chili powder

   Put all ingredients in blender or food processor. Blend until tomatoes and pepper are chopped coarse.

Tahini Dressing
   12 oz. of tahini sesame butter (raw)
   juice from 3 lemons
   1/2 c My-Protein
   dash of garlic, cayenne, kelp

   Mix well in blender. Keep refrigerated. Delicious over brown rice, noodles, salads, and soups, or as spread for sandwiches and steamed vegetables.

Special Sauce for Steamed Vegetables
   a handful of sunflower seed sprouts
   a handful of buckwheat sprouts
   1/2 avocado
   1/2 c lemon juice
   4 T sesame tahini
   4 T My-Protein
   garlic, vegetable seasoning, cayenne

   Blend and pour over steamed vegetables.

Healthful Green Dressing
    juice from 2 lemons
    1 c of water
    1 red onion
    fresh green chilies, seeds removed
    1 small bunch cilantro
    1 pinch cayenne,
    2 cloves garlic
    1 small bunch parsley

Blend until chopped coarse and use as salad dressing or turn into Wholly Guacamole.

Wholly Guacamole
    2 medium avocados, ripe

Smash avocado with fork, mix in Healthful Green Dressing. Serve on top of a vegetable salad, in place of salad dressing, or as a dip for celery stalks, or serve over noodles or rice.

Healthful Mayonnaise
Soak overnight:
    1 c of raw cashews in 1/3 c water.

Grind cashews in the blender and add the juice of one lemon, garlic, and cayenne. Store in a jar and serve as mayonnaise.

Chinese Ginger Sauce

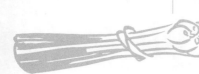

    2 cloves garlic
    2 green onions, chopped
    2 c water
    2 T arrowroot dissolved in 4 T water
    1 t oil
    1 T ginger, minced
    1 T olive oil
    4 T My-Protein

Sauté garlic, ginger, and onion in a little water. Add remaining water. Bring to a boil. Add My-Protein. Stir in arrowroot to thicken mixture, and add oil. Serve over steamed vegetables, tofu, or rice.

11 Salads

Salads contain lots of enzymes, vitamins, and minerals. They are very nutritional, easy to prepare, and fun to decorate.

Vegetables

Eat a large variety of the following vegetables daily: alfalfa and other sprouts, artichoke, arugula, asparagus, beets, broccoli, Brussels sprouts, cabbage (red or green), carrots, cauliflower, celery, chard, corn, cucumber, dill, eggplant, garlic, kale, kohlrabi, lettuce (Bibb, leaf, romaine—not iceberg), okra, onions, parsley, parsnips, peas, peppers, radish, scallions, spinach, string beans, squash, tomatoes, and zucchini.

Summer Green Salad

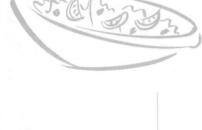

In a jar, shake well:
4 T oil
1/3 c lemon juice
dash Bio-Salt
1/4 c basil, finely chopped
1/8 c fresh dill, finely chopped

In a large salad bowl, layer:
4 c lettuce, spinach, and/or chard, torn into small pieces
1 c mustard greens, torn into small pieces
1 large tomato, cut into wedges
4 scallions, diced
1 1/2 c mushrooms, sliced thin
1 avocado, diced
1/2 c almonds, soaked 24 hours and cut in half

Pour dressing over salad and toss.

Avocado Salad

In a medium-sized salad bowl, layer:
1 avocado, cut into cubes
2 tomatoes, cut into chunks
1 bell pepper, cut in short slivers
1 c mushrooms, sliced
1/2 c sunflower seeds, soaked 12 hours

Pour dressing over salad and toss.

Gourmet Cold Salad

Grind in blender or food processor:
2 pkg frozen peas
2 green onions
4 fresh small carrots
1/3 cup tahini dressing

Mix to make into a thick paste. Serve a scoop over a lettuce leaf, pour dressing over, or fill a whole wheat pita pocket as a sandwich.

Healthy Living, A Holistic Guide

Salad Suggestions

It is a good idea to keep marinated veggies in the refrigerator to spruce up an ordinary salad. Vegetables should be very lightly steamed before putting in a vinaigrette (preferred substitute is lemon or lime juice). A good rule of thumb is 5 minutes, but this does vary. Suggested vinaigrette vegetables: string beans, cauliflower, broccoli, asparagus, etc.

Here is a quick list of some of the simpler but very tasty salads.

1. **Beets with Cloves**
   Steam beets. Drain. Slice in chunks. Marinate with ground cloves, oil, vinegar, and lime juice.

2. **Sprouts**
   Raw sprouts with lime juice, pepper, dried tomatoes, onions, and a dash of My-Protein.

3. **Grated Carrots**
   Raw, grated carrots marinated in orange and lime juices and sprinkled with cinnamon.

4. **Celery**
   Celery and lime juice with a dash of Healthful Mayonnaise.

5. **Diced Pineapple and Shredded Cabbage**
   Diced pineapple, shredded cabbage, lime juice, and raisins.

6. **Watercress and Mushrooms**
   Watercress and mushrooms in vinaigrette.

7. **Sliced Cucumber**
   Sliced cucumbers with dill weed and lime juice.

8. **Steamed Carrots**
   Steamed carrots with dill weed, lemon, or lime juice.

9. **Jicama**
   Jicama slices, sprinkled with lime juice and paprika.

10. **Rice and Lentil Salad**
    Toss leftover cooked rice or leftover cooked lentils with chopped raw onions, chopped tomatoes, and enough vinaigrette to flavor.

Fresh Corn Salad

Slice corn kernels off of the cob. Boil until tender. (If corn is very fresh, use it raw.) Drain well. Toss with chopped tomatoes, onions, parsley, and several finely chopped jalapeno chilies and the vinegar marinade. Also excellent with cold beans tossed in it.

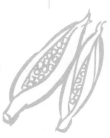

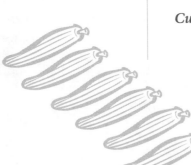

Cucumber Salad

6 cucumbers
2 cloves garlic, crushed
1/4 t tumeric (optional)
8 oz. kefir
1 T dill weed
2 T lemon or lime juice

Peel cucumbers and score. Slice thinly in rounds and marinate in mixture of kefir, garlic, dill weed, and lime juice. You may add tumeric for an interesting flavor, but it will color the mixture yellow.

Potato Salad

6 baked or broiled potatoes, diced
2 grated carrots
1 c diced celery
2 T finely diced onions
2 t celery seed
1 package of fresh or frozen peas, cooked
1/3 c chopped parsley
3 T of lime
1 t mustard powder
1 t rosemary
6 T Healthful Mayonnaise
6 T Healthful Green Dressing

Mix all ingredients and chill well before serving.

Spaghetti Squash Salad

1 spaghetti squash (about 2 1/2 lb)
8 cherry tomatoes, quartered
1 green bell pepper, chopped
4 scallions, sliced
1 c Wholly Guacamole

Preheat oven to 350 degrees. Prick squash with fork and bake for 45 minutes to 1 hour, until shell is easily depressed when touched with spoon. Cut squash in half, and remove seeds and stringy flesh. With a fork, gently scrape remaining flesh to remove spaghetti-like strands of squash. In a large salad bowl, combine squash, tomatoes, green peppers, and scallions. Toss Wholly Guacamole and season to taste.

Zucchini Salad

3 zucchinis
dash Bio-Salt and cayenne
few leaves of lettuce
1 tomato, chopped
2 T parsley, chopped
1 onion sliced
4 T olives
1 clove garlic, minced
2 carrots, shredded
3 T olive oil
6 radishes, sliced
1 cucumber, sliced

Lightly steam zucchini. Let it cool. Then chop zucchini and place it in a large mixing bowl. Add tomatoes, onions, and garlic, and combine gently. Add olive oil, Bio-Salt, and cayenne. Mix and refrigerate for 2 hours. To serve, line a serving platter with lettuce leaves, and scoop the zucchini mixture on top. Arrange carrots, radishes, and cucumbers around the edges.

Ginger Salad

2 c broccoli, chopped
3 c carrots, shredded
1 red pepper, sliced
1 sweet potato, cooled and cubed
2 t ginger powder
4 T lemon juice
1 c raisins
1/2 c Healthful Mayonnaise

Chop broccoli and shred carrots. Add sweet potatoes and pepper. Place them in large bowl and toss with the lemon juice. Toss the vegetables, ginger, mayonnaise, and raisins together.

Antipasto Salad

1 lb firm tofu, diced
1 c celery sliced
1/2 c mushrooms, sliced
1/2 red pepper, sliced
2 medium tomatoes, chopped
6 T Wholly Guacamole

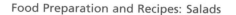

Mix the tofu and vegetables in a large bowl. Pour dressing and mix gently. Marinate in the refrigerator for 1 hour before serving.

Tomato Salad

1 onion, sliced
1/4 c apple cider vinegar
6 T olive oil
6 medium tomatoes, thickly sliced
6 oz. goat cheese (grated)

Place onions in a mixing bowl. In a saucepan, bring the vinegar just to a boil. Pour it over the onions. Let it sit until it cools. When cool, drain the vinegar, and blend the olive oil and Healthful Green Dressing. Place tomato slices on each serving plate. Arrange the onions on top of the tomatoes and sprinkle with cheese. Serve 1 T of Healthful Green Dressing and olive oil over each tomato.

Salad Florentine

3 c Boston lettuce
3 c spinach
4 potatoes, cooked, cooled, and cubed
2 c of green beans, cooked
1 c carrots, cooked, cooled, and cubed
1 c cherry tomatoes, halved
1 sliced and peeled cucumber
1 c red bell pepper strips
1/2 c olives

On a large serving plate, arrange lettuce and spinach leaves. Top with rows of potatoes, green beans, carrots, cucumbers, and bell peppers. Add olives and tomatoes. Serve with Wholly Guacamole Dressing.

Beans-Vegetable Salad

6 c escarole
2 c romaine
2 c white beans, cooked
2 c red beans, cooked
1 1/2 c diced celery
1 1/2 c cherry tomato, halved
1 c sliced zucchini
1/2 sliced onion
1/2 c fresh cilantro, chopped
1/2 c fresh parsley, chopped

In a big salad bowl, mix all ingredients. Add "Kelp from the Sea" Dressing.

Cooked Beet Salad

6 beets
1 carrot
1/4 cabbage

Steam beets; then cool. Scoop out centers. Shred cabbage and carrot, and mix with chopped beet centers. Mix with tahini dressing. Fill beet cups with mixture and chill. Serve on spinach leaves.

Rice Salad

1 c firm tofu, mashed
5 T My-Protein
1/2 c fresh parsley, chopped
2 c brown rice, cooked
1 yam, cubed
1 c broccoli
1 c water
1 c cauliflower

Steam yam, cauliflower, and broccoli until tender. Set aside. Mix rice with vegetables. Blend tofu with tahini dressing, water, and parsley in small saucepan. Heat for 5 minutes. Let it cool, and pour it over rice and vegetables. Chill and serve.

Winter Salad

Dressing—In a bowl, whip together with wire whisk:
4 T olive oil
1 T dill seed
1/4 c lemon juice
dash Bio-Salt

Pour dressing over 1/2 lb tofu, cut into cubes. Marinate for 1 hour or more, stirring occasionally.

Salad—In a large salad bowl, toss:
2 1/2 c cabbage, finely shredded
1 1/2 c carrots, grated
3/4 c radish, red and/or daikon, sliced thin
1/2 c onions, diced
1 tomato, cut
1/2 c sunflower seeds, soaked 12 hours

Pour the tofu/marinade over salad, and toss.

Spinach Tofu Salad

Dressing—In a jar, shake well:
4 T olive oil
2 T My-Protein
4 T lemon juice
1 t curry powder

Pour dressing over 1/2 lb tofu, cut into cubes. Marinate for 1 hour or more, stir occasionally

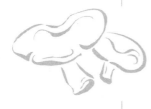

Salad—In a large bowl, toss:
5 c spinach, torn into small pieces
1 1/2 c mushrooms, sliced thin and halved
1 c mung bean sprouts
3/4 c red radish and/or daikon, sliced
4 scallions, diced

Pour marinated tofu over salad and toss.

12 Soups

Nothing like it on a cold day! So easy to prepare. Cook some extra and save it in your freezer.

Cleansing Mixed-Green Soup

1 small bunch greens of your choice
1/4 head red cabbage, shredded
1 small bunch of turnip greens
1 carrot scraped and diced
1/4 t fresh cracked pepper
1 small zucchini, diced
1 stalk celery, chopped
1 medium turnip, diced
1 small rutabaga, diced
1/4 t marjoram
1/4 t oregano
dash cayenne
1 medium beet, diced
1 onion, diced
1/2 lb fresh broccoli
3 qt water
1 bay leaf
1/4 t basil

Steam the following vegetables: Place the turnip, rutabaga, carrot, and beet in a deep soup pot with water. Simmer, covered, until the vegetables are partially tender. Then add all of the remaining ingredients and simmer, covered, for approximately 4 minutes. Place steamed vegetables and water in a blender, add My-Protein to taste, and serve. Serves 8 to 10 people.

Susana's Super Soup

1/2 potato
1/2 carrot
1/2 onion
1/2 sweet potato

Steam the vegetables. When almost done, add beet leaves, zucchini, celery. Blend steamed vegetables and water until slightly puréed. Add My-Protein, olive oil, garlic, kelp, and cayenne to season.

Winter Hearty Soup

1/2 c white lima beans
1/2 c green peas

Soak overnight and drain. Add fresh water and then add the following:
1 sweet potato, diced
1 large onion, chopped

1 bunch cilantro and parsley
1 c carrot pulp

Cook slowly. Add My-Protein, garlic, kelp, and cayenne to season.

Quick Energy Soup

In blender, place the following ingredients (all raw):
1 1/2 c water
1 medium organic carrot, chopped
1 organic apple, cored and chopped
1/2 medium onion
1 small handful of dulse (purplish seaweed)

Blend for about 15 seconds, and then add:
1 medium zucchini, chopped
1/2 stalk of celery
1/4 t basil leaves
3 T My-Protein
dash cayenne

Blend for 15 seconds, and then add:
1 medium avocado
1 small handful freshly cut buckwheat lettuce
1 small handful freshly cut sunflower greens

Blend for 15 seconds and serve.

Asparagus Soup

1 lb asparagus, chopped
2 T olive oil
1 medium onion, diced
2 celery stalks, diced
1 medium potato, diced
1/4 t tarragon
1/2 t parsley
1/4 t rosemary
2 qt water
dash of Bio-Salt and cayenne pepper
1/4 c chopped cilantro

In a large soup pot, sauté the onions and celery until tender—3 to 5 minutes. Add the asparagus, potato, cayenne and herbs. Then add enough water to cover the vegetables. Bring to a boil, lower heat, and simmer for

25 to 30 minutes until the vegetables are tender. Remove from heat, and cool for 5 minutes. Purée the vegetables in small batches in a blender, returning each batch to the soup pot. Serve immediately with a garnish of chopped cilantro.

Bean Soup

1 onion, chopped
1 carrot, chopped
1 stalk celery, chopped
1 T olive oil
2 c cooked beans
8 c water
fresh basil
1/2 t oregano
pinch Bio-Salt
pinch cayenne
pinch garlic powder

Sauté onion, carrot, and celery in a little water. Add 1 cup of beans and water. Purée the remaining beans and 1 cup of water in a blender. Stir in the remaining ingredients. Bring to a boil, lower heat, and simmer for 15 minutes. Serve and add olive oil and My-Protein.

13 Main Dishes

Tofu: "Meat Without the Bone"
Low in calories, high in good-quality protein, and rich in
both calcium and iron. Ideal for weight watchers. An 8-oz.
serving contains 147 to 164 calories.

Tofu Spread

12 oz. tofu
1/3 c almond butter (optional)
1 1/2 bananas
2 T lemon juice
2 T honey

Combine all ingredients in a blender and purée until smooth. Serve on a seven-grain bread and top with nuts, raisins, or sliced bananas.

Tofu-Avocado Spread

8 oz. tofu
1 avocado
2 T Healthful Mayonnaise
1 pinch cayenne, garlic, and kelp
2 T My-Protein

Mix all ingredients in blender. Serve with all raw vegetables.

Tofu, Carrot, Raisin, and Walnut Salad

6 oz. tofu, well drained
1 c grated carrots
1/2 c raisins
1/2 c walnuts, diced
1 1/2 T miso
2 t honey
1 t lemon juice
2 T sesame butter
4 lettuce leaves

Wrap tofu in a cloth towel, squeeze the water, and let it sit for 15 minutes until firm. Mash well. Combine with rest of ingredients and mix well. Serve on lettuce or in sandwiches.

Tofu-Pita Pizza

Use tofu, soy cheese, fresh tomatoes, cayenne, garlic, kelp, fresh oregano, and basil.

Stuff pita with all ingredients and bake in oven for 15 minutes.

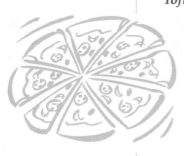

Tofu and Onions

onions
tofu
My-Protein
garlic powder
cayenne
kelp

Chop onions and sauté in water. Chop tofu into cubes and add to onions. Add garlic, cayenne, and kelp; cover and simmer. Allow to cook for a few minutes; remove from heat. Add My-Protein and olive oil, and serve over steamed vegetables.

Pasta

Pasta is low in calories and fat and is rich in complex carbohydrates. Pasta is easy to make and is used in an endless variety of recipes. Read label for whole-grain pastas. No white, enriched, or bleached flour.

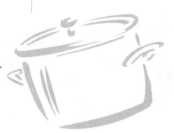

Boil pasta according to instructions and drain.
1. Add olive oil and My-Protein. Season with cayenne, garlic, kelp, and chopped cilantro.
2. Add tahini dressing.
3. Add Healthful Tomato Sauce.
4. Add Wholly Guacamole.

Pasta
Look for artichoke, brown rice, oat, corn, spelt, whole durham flour, quinoa, etc.

Pasta Deliciosa

Season with the following variations:
2 T Wholly Guacamole
2 T Tahini Dressing
1 T olive oil
3 T My-Protein
1 pinch cayenne, garlic, and kelp
2 T nut milk

Stir ingredients together and serve.

Healthful Tomato Sauce

In a pan, boil 1/2 cup water and sauté the following:
4 large red onions, chopped
6 carrots, grated
4 fresh tomatoes, chopped

3 zucchini, chopped
1 red bell pepper, chopped
3 cloves of garlic
1/2 c parsley, chopped
1/2 c cilantro, chopped

Cover and simmer for an hour. At serving time, add the following:
2 T olive oil
2 T My-Protein
1 pinch of cayenne, garlic, and kelp

Pour over noodles.

Pasta Al Olio (Garlic-Oil-Parsley)
1 package (1 lb) pasta
6 T olive oil
3 cloves garlic
whole cayenne peppers
1 bunch parsley, as finely cut as possible
Vegan parmesan cheese, freshly grated

Cook pasta and drain. While pasta is cooking, sauté garlic pieces and cayenne in olive oil until golden brown. Add sautéed garlic, cayenne, and parsley to drained pasta and toss. Sprinkle with Vegan parmesan cheese.

Papaya Noodles
1 package (1lb) medium-sized pasta
6 T olive oil
dash cayenne
1 papaya, peeled, seeded, and chopped
1 c cherry tomatoes, halved
1 bunch green onions, thinly sliced
1 yellow bell pepper, seeded and chopped
1 cucumber, quartered lengthwise and sliced
6 T rice vinegar
1 small jalapeno pepper, finely minced
2 T chopped fresh cilantro or parsley

Cook pasta. Drain and transfer to medium-sized bowl; add oil and season with cayenne to taste. Cool to room temperature. Add papaya, tomatoes, sliced green onions, bell pepper, and cucumber, and toss together. In small bowl, combine vinegar, jalapeno pepper, and cilantro. Add to pasta and toss to combine. Refrigerate 1 to 2 hours or until chilled. To serve, garnish with green onion brushes.

Basil-Pesto Pasta

    3 cloves garlic
    2 c fresh basil
    1/4 c pine nuts
    1/4 c olive oil
    1/3 c goat cheese
    1 box pasta

Blend garlic, basil, pine nuts, and oil for 2 to 3 minutes. Add cheese and blend for 1 more minute. Boil pasta and drain. Add pesto mixture and serve. Make extra pesto sauce and refrigerate.

Bow Ties with Greens and Mushrooms

    1 package (8 oz.) bow tie noodles
    3 T olive oil
    3 green onions, chopped
    3/4 c sliced mushrooms
    1 rib celery, thinly sliced
    dash finely grated, peeled ginger root
    1 pound kale, spinach, or other dark leafy green, rinsed (tough stalks removed and broken into small pieces)
    dash Bio-Salt
    3/4 c water
    2 T arrowroot powder
    1/4 c cold water
    1/4 c grated goat cheese

Cook pasta and drain. Meanwhile, in large skillet over medium heat, heat oil. Add green onions, mushrooms, celery, and ginger. Cook 2 to 3 minutes, stirring constantly; do not brown. Add kale and 3/4 cup water. Cover; reduce heat to low, and cook about 15 minutes or until vegetables are tender-crisp. In small bowl, mix arrowroot powder with cold water; stir into vegetable mixture and cook just until heated through. To serve, toss vegetables with hot pasta in medium-sized bowl sprinkle with shredded goat cheese and Bio-Salt.

Anchovy Pasta

    1 package (1 lb) spaghetti
    1 T olive oil
    3 garlic cloves, thinly sliced
    1/4 T red pepper flakes
    6 anchovy fillets, finely chopped
    1 jar (6 1/2 oz.) oil-cured olives, pitted
    3 large, ripe tomatoes, chopped

Use your imagination to mix an endless variety of vegetables, grains, seeds, and nuts.

dash cayenne
fresh cilantro (optional)

Cook pasta; drain. Meanwhile, in large skillet over medium heat, heat oil. Stir in garlic, pepper flakes, and anchovies; cook 1 minute. Add olives and tomatoes; cook 8 to 10 minutes or until sauce thickens, stirring occasionally. Season with cayenne to taste. To serve, toss pasta with sauce in large bowl, garnish with cilantro and serve immediately.

Radish Leaf Delight Pasta
3 bunches radish leaves, washed well
1 package (8 oz.) linguini or other long, thin pasta
6 T olive oil
dash cayenne pepper and Bio-Salt
goat cheese, freshly grated

Cook pasta and radish leaves together; drain. Place back into the pan, add olive oil and cayenne pepper; toss to combine. Sprinkle with cheese.

Linguini with Broccoli and Feta
1 package (8 oz.) linguini or other long, thin pasta
2 bunches broccoli, cut into small florets and stems removed
2 T oil
2 large garlic cloves, minced
5 green onions, thinly sliced
1 1/2 T chopped fresh thyme or 1/2 tsp dried thyme leaves
4 oz. feta cheese or soft goat cheese
dash cayenne and Bio-Salt

Cook pasta; drain. Meanwhile, steam broccoli florets about 3 minutes or just until tender-crisp; set aside. In large skillet over medium-high heat, heat oil. Add garlic and green onions; cook about 1 minute or until tender but not brown, stirring often. Add thyme and reserved broccoli; cook 2 minutes longer, stirring often. Remove from heat; add feta cheese. Transfer mixture to large bowl; add hot pasta and toss together. To serve, season with cayenne to taste.

Summer Dream Pasta
1 bunch parsley, finely cut
4 tomatoes, cut into finger-tip-sized pieces
5-7 garlic cloves, finely cut
juice of 1 lemon
dash cayenne pepper and Bio-Salt

goat cheese, freshly grated
1 package (8 oz.) spaghetti or other pasta

Cook pasta; drain. While pasta is cooking, place lemon juice, cayenne pepper, Bio-Salt, garlic cloves, tomatoes, and parsley into a bowl and stir until well mixed. Add this mixture to drained pasta. Sprinkle with parmesan cheese. Serve hot or cold.

Lasagna

1 package De Boles Lasagna
1 package tofu
1 package soy cheese
1 package goat cheese

Boil noodles and drain carefully. In a rectangular pan, alternate: 1 layer Healthful Tomato Sauce, 1 layer lasagna noodles, 1 layer grated cheese and tofu. Continue layers until pan is almost full. Bake at 350 degrees for 30 minutes. Serve with green salad.

Other Dishes

Vegetable Loaf

carrots
broccoli
summer squash
jicama
cauliflower
cucumber
yellow squash
onion

Grate all raw vegetables above or add your own favorites (use amount of vegetables appropriate to your family size). In a bowl, combine enough cashew butter with a little tahini to make mixture stick together. You may want to add a bit of vegetable seasoning. Mix with grated vegetables. Press mixture into small individual loaf pans; turn out onto a plate lined with sprouts and sliced tomatoes.

Sunburgers

2 medium carrots, grated
1 onion, chopped fine
1 t parsley
1/2 c oatmeal
1/8 t sweet basil

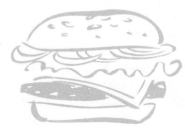

1 c celery, chopped fine
1 fresh tomato chopped
dash Bio-Salt
1 c sunflower seeds, ground

Mix all ingredients raw. Form into patties. Bake 30 minutes at 350 degrees. May need turning halfway through baking time.

Creamy Eggplant Casserole
2 large eggplants
3 c brown rice, cooked
1 green pepper
1 medium onion
2 c raw cashews
1 c water
dash Bio-Salt
1/2 t celery salt
1/4 t garlic salt
1/2 t sage
3 T parsley
2-4 almonds

Cube eggplant. Boil until tender (do not overcook). Chop pepper and onion and sauté over low heat in water. Whiz 1 c water into blender with cashews; blend until smooth. Drain eggplant and add onion and pepper. Stir until eggplant is slightly mashed. Add rice, nut mixture, and seasoning. Blend well. Pour into casserole, sprinkle with almonds, and bake for 1 hour at 325 degrees.

Millet Tomato Loaf
1 c millet, uncooked
1 c tomato juice
1 medium onion, quartered
dash Bio-Salt
1/2 c olives, chopped
1/2 t sage
1/2 t savory
5 c fresh tomatoes
1/2 c nuts or seeds

In a 2-quart casserole dish, combine 1 c tomato juice with millet and olives, and soak overnight. Blend smooth the remaining ingredients. Stir into casserole. Cover and bake at 350 degrees for 1 hour and 20 minutes. Remove from oven, take lid off, and let set 10 minutes before serving.

Split Pea Stew

    1 1/2 c dry split peas
    6 c water
    2 tomatoes, chopped
    1 red pepper, chopped
    1 onion, chopped
    2 cloves garlic, chopped
    1/4 c chopped parsley and cilantro
    2 c cubed sweet potatoes
    2 c carrot pulp
    2 c small broccoli florets
    chopped parsley for garnish
    4 T My-Protein

Soak peas overnight. Bring peas and soaking water to a boil. Add tomatoes. Simmer, covered, until peas are very soft (30 minutes). In a blender or food processor, purée pea mixture until smooth, adding a little extra water if necessary. Return puréed peas to a saucepan. Cover and keep warm.

In a large, deep pot, combine onion, garlic, parsley, cilantro, sweet potatoes, and the remaining 2 c water. Bring to a boil, reduce heat, and simmer 6 to 7 minutes. Add broccoli and carrots, and simmer another 6 to 8 minutes or until broccoli is tender. Add pea mixture, reduce heat to low, cover, and cook gently. Serve and garnish with parsley, cilantro, and My-Protein.

Zucchini Casserole with Grains

    For one large casserole, cook 1 c rice (or other grain) in 2 c water.
    2 zucchinis, sliced thinly
    1 eggplant, sliced thinly
    6 cloves garlic, crushed
    3/4 c raw almonds
    1 tomato, sliced in 1/2-inch circles
    sesame seeds, sunflower seeds
    oregano, basil, and parsley
    2 carrots, sliced in circles
    1 onion, sliced in circles
    1 c raw sliced celery
    1 c grated or cubed Tofurella

When all vegetables are sliced, steam each separately (or keep separate in a steamer) for approximately 5 minutes. Remove from heat. Lightly oil casserole dish. Put a thin layer of grain mixture on the bottom of the pan, and add successive layers of zucchini, onions, almonds and seeds, oregano, carrots, celery basil, parsley, and so on until top of casserole is reached. Top with sliced tomatoes and sprinkle with grated Tofurella and sesame seeds. Bake covered for 45 minutes at 450 degrees.

Sweet Potato Sticks
    2 large sweet potatoes
    1/2 c sesame seeds
    1 T sesame oil

Boil sweet potatoes until soft but not mushy. Let cool or refrigerate overnight. Peel and cut potatoes into pieces about 2 1/2" x 1/2". Roll potato sticks in sesame seeds, pressing to make seeds stick. Sauté in oil for 1 minute on each side, drain, and cool. Serve cool or broil briefly and serve hot.

Chop Suey

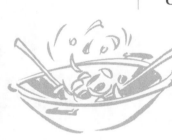

    2 zucchini
    2 yellow squash
    2 onions, chopped
    1 c sprouts (beans or lentils)
    3 celery stalks, sliced
    3 green onions, chopped
    3 c Chinese peas
    6 T olive oil
    5 T My-Protein

*Put 1/2 cup water in pan and heat. Add sliced zucchini squash, onions, celery, and Chinese peas. Sauté briefly at low heat. **Do not overcook**. Just before removing from fire, add sprouts. Turn off heat and let stand about 5 minutes. Now add olive oil and My-Protein. Serve over rice, garnish with green onions, and sprinkle with ground almonds.*

Baked Sweet Potatoes
    12 sweet potatoes
    1/2 c of nut milk
    3 apples, chopped
    1/2 c almonds, chopped

Boil sweet potatoes and let chill. Remove top lengthwise from each potato, cutting off no more then 1/4 of the potato. Scoop out insides of potatoes (do not break the skin). Place the contents in a blender, adding nut milk, apples, and almonds until you obtain a creamy consistency. Spoon mixture back into potatoes. Reheat on top rack of oven at 250 degrees for 45 minutes.

Sweet and Sour Cabbage
  1 carrot
  1 small cabbage
  2 apples
  2 T date crystals
  1/3 c lemon juice
  3 T olive oil
  1 pint water
  3 cloves
  dash Bio-Salt

Shred cabbage and carrot. Put 1/2 c water in sauce pan and add shredded vegetables. Shred apples, and mix with water, lemon juice, date crystals, Bio-Salt, and cloves. Pour over grated vegetables and cook at low temperature until tender. Now add olive oil and serve.

Vegetable Noodle Casserole
  1 package of De Boles noodles (8 oz.)
  4 c chopped vegetables:
    celery, onions, red peppers, water, chestnuts, parsley
  3 T olive oil
  3 c water
  3 T Tahini Dressing

Boil noodles until tender. Strain. Sauté vegetables (in a little water) until tender, add noodles, and stir lightly with a fork. Add remaining water, oil, and tahini dressing and serve.

Eggplant Spread
  1 eggplant
  1 onion
  1 c celery
  juice of 1 lemon
  dash Bio-Salt and cayenne
  2 T olive oil
  1/4 lb Grecian olives
  1 clove garlic

Bake eggplant. When done, remove peeling. Do not lose any of the juice while peeling. Mix all ingredients in a blender and chill. Use on toast, crackers, or cut vegetables.

Millet-Stuffed Onions

12 medium-sized onions
1/2 c millet, uncooked
2 1/2 c of water
dash Bio-Salt
2 cloves garlic, minced
1/2 c mushrooms, sliced
1/2 c celery, sliced
2 T olive oil
1/2 c chickpeas, cooked
1 c almonds, grated
2 t My-Protein
2 t lemon juice
parsley for garnish

Hollow out insides of onions with an apple core, leaving bottoms intact and reserving insides. Steam hollowed out onions until tender, reserving 3/4 cup of cooking liquid. Soak and cook millet. Remove from heat and let stand, covered, for 10 minutes. Fluff with a fork. Finely chop reserved onions. Sauté chopped onion, garlic, mushrooms, and celery for 15 minutes. Mix in millet and chickpeas for about 5 minutes. Fill onions with millet mixture. Crush almonds, My-Protein, and lemon juice in blender, and add reserved cooking liquid. Place mixture in a saucepan and heat, stirring constantly. Pour over stuffed onions, garnish, and serve.

Quinoa Casserole

1 c quinoa, uncooked
1 T olive oil
2 onions, thinly sliced
3 stalks celery, thinly sliced
1 c chickpeas, cooked
5 c water
dash Bio-Salt
2 c broccoli, chopped
parsley, minced, for garnish

Rinse and drain quinoa. Dry-roast quinoa in heavy skillet for 6 minutes, stirring constantly. Remove from heat. In 4 T of water, sautée onions. Add celery, stirring often, for about 5 minutes. Add chickpeas, water, and salt. Bring to a boil. Stir in quinoa and return to a boil. Reduce heat, cover, and simmer for 15 minutes. Add broccoli and continue to cook for 5 minutes. Add oil. While mixture is hot, press firmly into a 9-inch pan. Sprinkle with garnish, cut into squares, and serve.

Sun Seed Paté

In blender (nutrition center Vita Mix), blend until slightly chunky:
2 c sunflower, pumpkin, or sesame seeds (soaked)
1 c alfalfa, onion, and/or radish sprouts
3 scallions
2 stalks celery or cucumber
1/4 c fresh parsley
3 T lemon juice
1 T dried basil
3 t My-Protein
dash of cayenne

Put in a bowl and stir in 1/2 c carrots, grated. Decorate with sprigs of parsley and sprinkles of cayenne. Serve with sprouted wheat or rye crackers.

Falafel Patties

In Vita Mix blender, mix until smooth and creamy:
2 c garbanzo beans, soaked 48 hours
1/2 c sesame seeds, soaked 12 hours
1/2 c wheatberry sprouts
1/4 c fresh parsley
1 T curry powder
1 T basil
1 T cumin powder
2 T My-Protein
1/8 t cayenne

Form into 2-inch balls. Place in dehydrator for 4 to 6 hours or until a crust has formed on outside. The inside will be moist. Making Falafels: Place several patties on a grain crisp. Layer shredded lettuce and diced tomatoes and cucumber. Cover with Tahini Dressing and serve.

Croquettes

2 c lentil sprouts
1 clove garlic
1/4 T cumin
1 c seeds (make into cheese by soaking and grinding)
2 carrots grated
1/4 c scallion

Grind or mash lentils. Mix with other ingredients. Shape into croquettes and roll in poppy seeds.

Tabouli

    1 c cracked wheat
    1 c finely chopped green onions, with tops
    3 c fresh parsley, chopped
    3 c of fresh cilantro, chopped
    4 finely chopped tomatoes
    1/2 c of lemon juice
    1/2 c of olive oil
    Add cayenne, garlic, and kelp

Soak cracked wheat overnight. Mix all remaining ingredients together. Add to soaked wheat. Allow to set for 3 hours so wheat can absorb flavors, and serve.

Tabouli Casserole

Soak 1 c millet and 1 c cracked wheat overnight. Add remaining ingredients from previous recipe. Cook and serve.

Tasty Legumes Recipe

Soak 2 c overnight (garbanzos, lentils, or any type of beans). Drain water and add fresh water; cook for 2 hours at low heat. Add while cooking:
    1/2 c parsley, chopped
    1/2 c cilantro, chopped
    1 c onions, chopped
    1 c carrots, chopped
    3 cloves garlic

When ready to serve, add:
    2 T olive oil
    2 T My-Protein
    1 pinch cayenne, garlic, and kelp

Serve with brown rice or millet.

Neurofuzzy Rice Cooker

Multi-purpose cooker for rice and other grains, steamed vegetables, and casseroles. Features:

- Nonstick inner pan (not aluminum or Teflon)
- Easy to operate and never burns a meal
- Digital timer allows programming up to 13 hours in advance
- Fast-cooking
- Prepares delicious casseroles in just minutes

- When food is perfectly cooked, it automatically stops cooking and switches to "warm."

Rice Cooker Operating Instructions

1. Plug Rice Cooker in.
2. Select the type of grain by pressing the **Menu** button.

   Types of Grain
   Regular—for brown rice, mixed rice, quinoa
   Softer—for white rice, porridge
   Harder—for fried rice, whole wheat, millet
3. Measure 1 c of grain and 2 c of water (rice or any other grain). You can add a portion of fresh chopped veggies or a packet of frozen veggies.
   Do not add any more water.
   Press the **Cooking/Reheat** button.
4. Grain machine will switch to "keep warm" when finished.

To program your cooker when you want your rice to be ready at a later time:

1. Plug Rice Cooker in.
2. Press the **Timer** button (it will display 6:00 A.M.)
3. Press the **Menu** button to select what type of grain (regular, hard, soft)
4. Press **Hour** and **Minute** keys to display what time you want your rice to be ready (example, 6:30 P.M.)
5. When you press the **Cooking/Reheating** button, the rice cooker will automatically switch itself on at the time you have set.
6. When rice is finshied, it will switch to the "keep warm" mode.

Rice Cooker Recipes

Plain Grain

1 cup grain: millet, quinoa, brown rice, whole-wheat kernels, or steel-cut oat (Two different grains can be mixed.)

Add 2 c water, turn switch on "regular." When cooking is perfectly done, cooker will switch to warm.

Potato Casserole

3 onions (sliced)
3 bell peppers (sliced)
4 potatoes (sliced)
4 sweet potatoes (sliced)

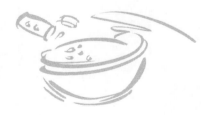

1 c water
1/2 c Tahini Dressing or Healthful Green Dressing.

Place in cooker half the onions and peppers and half the potatoes and sweet potatoes. Add the remaining onions, peppers, and potatoes. Add 1 c water. Add 1/2 c Tahini Dressing or Healthful Green Dressing. Turn cooker on "regular." Cook for 20 minutes, unplug cooker, and add My-Protein, cayenne, Bio-Salt, etc.

Fast and Tasty Paella

1 c grain
2 c water
1 pkg frozen vegetables
(green peas, corn, or mixed)
You may add 1/2 to 1/3 c Healthful Green Dressing, Tahini Dressing, or nut milk
You may also add fresh vegetables, chopped into bite-size pieces: onions, tomatoes, zucchini, carrots, sweet potatoes, etc.
You may also add:
chicken, fish, or tofu (chopped into bite-size pieces)

Turn switch to "regular." When cooking is done, the cooker automatically switches to warm.

Vegetable Soup

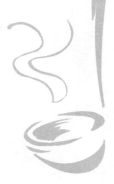

2 qt hot water
3 c mixed chopped vegetables: onion, celery, potatoes, parsley, garlic, zucchini, etc.

Cook on "regular" for 20 minutes. Unplug cooker, and serve with My-Protein and cayenne.

14 Healthful Sweets

Use healthful ingredients (no white flour or sugar please).

Start experimenting with your palate.

Your family will be glad you did!

Baked Apples and Pears

Filling:
1/2 c dried apricots, chopped
1 c almonds ground
1 T honey
1/2 tsp cinnamon
1/2 banana
juice of 1 orange
juice of 1 lemon

To prepare filling: Soak dried apricots in warm water until soft, about 15 minutes. Combine apricots with remaining filling ingredients in mixing bowl. Set aside.

To assemble: Preheat oven to 400 degrees. Core apples and pears, and sprinkle with a little lemon juice. Press filling into cored area of each fruit. Place in lightly greased baking dish. Bake for 20 minutes or until tender but still firm. Remove fruit and let cool.

Tofu-Pita Dessert

1 lb cake tofu
2 T rice syrup or maple syrup
1 T almond butter
4 to 6 pita pockets

Squeeze excess water out of the tofu. Blend tofu, rice syrup, and almond butter together. Fill pita pockets and lightly bake for a few minutes.

Fruit Salad

1 cup freshly squeezed orange juice
juice of 1/2 a lemon
2 apples
2 pears
2 peaches
2 bananas
1/2 pound grapes

Combine the orange juice and lemon juice in a large bowl. Add each fruit as you cut it, so that the juice in the bowl will keep it from discoloring. Cover the bowl with plastic wrap, and chill in the refrigerator for at least 2 hours before serving.

Tofurella Cheesecake

Filling:
2 lb tofurella
1 t vanilla
3 t lemon juice
1/3 c almond butter
6 T rice bran syrup
dash cinnamon
Crust:
1 1/2 c of granola, crushed
3/4 c graham cracker crumbs
1 T melted raw butter
2 T rice bran syrup
apple juice to moisten

Preheat oven to 350 degrees. Pulverize the granola and graham crackers together into very fine crumbs in a mixing bowl. Melt butter and rice syrup together over low heat. Add to the crumbs just enough apple juice to make mixture hold together. Press the crumb mixture evenly into a greased 9-inch pie pan. Bake for 10 minutes, remove, and cool completely. Reduce oven temperature to 325 degrees. Purée all of the filling ingredients in a blender until smooth. Pour the filling mixture into the crust, and bake at 325 degrees for 30 minutes. Turn the oven off, but leave the cheesecake in the oven for another 30 minutes. Serve.

Sesame Crackers

2 c of water
1 1/2 c oil
2 t Bio-Salt
8 c whole-wheat flour
2 c sesame seeds

Blend water, oil, and salt. Combine flour and sesame seeds with this mixture. Knead a little. Let rest 10 minutes. Roll out the dough and cut into cookie-size pieces. Bake at 350 degrees for 15 to 30 minutes.

Peanut Butter Apple Sandwiches

1 medium apple
2 T peanut butter or almond butter
2 T soft or regular tofu, well drained
1 T orange juice

Peel the apple while it is still whole. Cut apple crosswise into four to six slices. Cut out the core with a knife to make rings. In a bowl, mash together tofu and peanut butter until almost smooth, then spread on one apple slice to make a sandwich. Repeat with remaining slices.

Barbecued Peaches with Cream

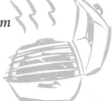

6 fresh peaches—ripe
1 T melted butter
dash cinnamon

Wash peaches and cut in half. Remove pits. Brush with melted butter and barbeque a few minutes on each side. To serve, add one of the following dressings.

Mix in blender: 3 oz. kefir or yogurt and 1/4 c almonds

Almond Cream

1 c almonds, soaked 48 hours
1/2 c dates, pitted
1 t vanilla extract
1 banana
1 c water
2 T lemon juice

In a blender, blend until smooth and creamy.

Tofu Cream

1 lb firm tofu
2 bananas
2 T honey
2 T lemon juice
2 T tahini or almond butter (optional)
1/2 t vanilla

In a blender, blend until smooth and creamy.

Healthful Birthday Treat—Raggedy Ann Fruit Salad

bananas—Arms
coconut—Hair
pears—Face
pineapple round—Chest
red cherries—Feet
red hots (candies)—Nose, Eyes, Buttons
fruit salad covered with lettuce—Skirt

Apricot Pie

Filling:
In bowl, soak for 6 hours:
2 c apricots, cut in half
3 c water

Blend in blender until smooth and creamy:
1 c almonds, soaked 48 hours
10 dates
2 T psyllium seed husks
Water from soaked apricots

Place in bowl and stir in soaked apricots.

Pie Shell:
Blend until smooth and creamy:
2 c almonds, not soaked
1/4 c raisins
1/2 t cinnamon
1-2 T water

Press pie shell into a 9-inch baking pan. Pour apricot filling into pie shell. Chill and serve.

15 Herbs

The following information is for educational purposes only. It is not intended to replace the services of any health professional.

Historic Uses of Nature's Herbs

Alfalfa
For pituitary gland, arthritis, chlorophyll, highly nutritive, alkalizes body rapidly, detoxifies body and liver.

Algin
Detoxification, absorbs heavy metals such as lead and cadmium, able to remove any radiation from the body.

Barberry Bark
Laxative, typhoid, jaundice, improves appetite.

Bayberry
Has been used for congestion in the nose and sinuses. It is extremely good for all female organs.

Bee Pollen
Energy food and allergies.

Black Cohosh
Female estrogen, menstrual cramps, high blood pressure, spinal meningitis, poisonous bites, relieves childbirth pain at delivery.

Black Currant Oil
Builds blood, high in vitamin C, highly alkalizing, one of the highest sources of GLA.

Black Walnut
Cleanses parasites, TB, expels tapeworms, diarrhea.

Blessed Thistle
Strengthens the heart and lungs, takes oxygen to the brain.

Blue Cohosh
Regulates menstrual flow, makes childbirth easier, whooping cough, bronchial mucus, palpitations, high blood pressure and spasms.

Buckthorn
Rheumatism, gout, dropsy, skin disease.

Burdock
Acne, arthritis, boils, blood purifier, cleansing, skin diseases, eczema.

Butcher's Broom

Varicose veins, hemorrhoids, anti-inflammatory, phlebitis, helps kidneys.

Capsicum

Catalyst for all herbs, stops internal bleeding, circulation, use with lobelia for nerves.

Cascara Sagrada

Chronic constipation, gall stones, increases secretion of bile.

Catnip

Convulsions in children, sleep aid, soothing to nerves, insanity.

Chamomile

Nerves, toothache, helps stop smoking and use of alcohol, muscle pain.

Chaparral

Cleanser, arthritis, blood purifier, acne and boils.

Chickweed

Bronchial cleanser, "eats" carbohydrates, deafness, peritonitis.

Comfrey

Blood cleanser, ulcers, stomach, kidneys, bowel.

Cornsilk

Used for kidney and bladder trouble, trouble with prostate gland in urinating, also for painful urination, and to prevent bed wetting.

Damiana

Sexual impotency, reproductive organs, overcome loss of nerves, energy to limbs.

Dandelion

Blood builder and purifier, liver cleanser, very good for anemia.

Dong Quai

Female correctional problems, blood pressure, liver and blood cleanser.

Echinacea

Antispasmodic, prevents infection from spreading, skin problems, lymph glands, circulation, fevers.

Evening Primrose Oil

Weight loss, high blood pressure, eczema, hot flashes, multiple sclerosis, arthritis, alcoholism.

Eyebright

Aids vision, uppermost parts of the throat as far as the windpipe.

False Unicorn

Miscarriage, problems with the female reproductive system, sterility, diabetes.

Fennel

Has been used to eliminate colic in babies, helps kill appetite, aids digestion when uric acid is the problem.

Fenugreek

Healing fevers, lubricates intestines, useful for the eyes, moves mucus.

Garlic

Has been used to emulsify cholesterol and loosen it from arterial walls, effective in arresting intestinal putrefaction and infection.

Ginger

Stimulates circulation.

Ginseng

Male hormone, longevity, prostate, stomach problems.

Golden Seal

Antibiotic, acts as insulin, cleanser, morning sickness, cure-all type herb.

Gotu Kola

Mental troubles, blood pressure, energy, depression, longevity, strengthens the heart, memory, and brain, nervous breakdowns.

Grapevine

Smog, diuretic.

Hawthorn Berries

Has been used to dilate coronary blood vessels mildly and restore heart muscle wall.

Hops

Insomnia, restlessness, shock, decreases desire for alcohol.

Ho-Shu-Wu

Longevity herb.

Horsetail

Has been used as a diuretic, heavy in silica, helps with kidney stones.

Hydrangea

Gall stones, kidney stones, bladder, diuretic.

Juniper Berries

Has been used for kidney or bladder problems related to pancreas and adrenal glands.

Kelp

Thyroid, arteries, nails, hair falling out, cleanses radiation from body.

Licorice Root

Natural cortisone, hypoglycemia, adrenal glands, stress, voice, colds.

Lobelia

Strong relaxant, emetic in large amounts, asthma, angina pectoris, epilepsy, strengthens muscle action, weak heart, use with capsicum.

Mullein

Has been used for breathing problems, hay fever, pain killer, glandular swelling.

Pau D'Arco

Cancer (all types), diabetes, Hodgkin's disease, leukemia, blood builder, psoriasis, ulcers, and more.

Psyllium

Excellent colon cleanser, creates bulk, anti-intoxication.

Red Clover

Blood purifier, relaxes the nerves and entire system.

Rosehips

Has been used as an infection fighter, also used as a stress herb.

Sage

Used to prevent night sweats, expels worms in children and adults, stops bleeding of wounds and cleans old ulcers and sores.

Sarsaparilla

Male hormone, rheumatism, gout, psoriasis, antidote for poison.

Skullcap

Nerve tonic, rabies, hysteria, migraines, strengthens heart.

Slippery Elm

Inflamed mucous membranes of the stomach, bowels, kidneys.

Spirulina

Energy, RNA-DNA balancer, high protein, kills appetite.

Uva Ursi

Diabetes, kidneys, hemorrhoids, spleen, liver, pancreas, gonorrhea.

Valerian Root.

Nervous disorders, headache, muscle twitching, spasms. Promotes sleep.

White Oak Bark

Decongestant, blood purifier, asthma, hay fever, flu.

Yucca

Has been used for rheumatoid and osteoid forms of arthritis.

16 Home Remedies

You will be surprised to learn of the effects of some of the most common foods, such as garlic, onions, grapefruit, capsicum (cayenne), lemons, chlorophyll, and vitamin C.

Natures Antibiotics

Onions and garlic, along with vitamin C, are the most important antibiotics in nature.

Onion and Garlic Tea

Cut three large onions or two large bulbs (not cloves) of garlic crosswise into a quart and a half of water (they need not be peeled). Cook until tender (do not use aluminum cookware). Strain and drink a cup of this tea every 20 minutes. Onion or garlic tea is almost tasteless but very effective. Cayenne makes it more effective, and tomato juice may be added.

Grapefruit—Antibiotic, Bacteriostatic

The bitter tea of grapefruit is as effective as quinine, with no side effects. It relieves aching and discomfort associated with acute infectious diseases. Cooking onions or garlic with the grapefruit makes it doubly effective. You cannot make the grapefruit tea taste worse by adding onions or garlic, so why not combine them?

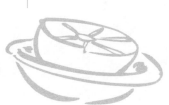

Grapefruit and Garlic Tea:

Remove the yellow peel of two grapefruits with a potato peeler. Cut the fruit thinly, with two large bulbs of garlic, into a quart and a half of water. Cook until very bitter, about 20 minutes. Drink a cup of this tea every 20 minutes, and by the time the quart and a half of tea is gone, the infection is usually gone too. I use this along with enemas.

Peach leaf and yarrow are, like grapefruit, as effective as quinine, and may be substituted for grapefruit if the fruit is not available.

Capsicum-Cayenne, Red Pepper—Antibiotic, Bacteriostatic

Cayenne equalizes the circulation and has an influence on the whole system. It may be added to the teas mentioned above. It promotes elimination through the skin when sweat baths or Epsom salt pouring baths are taken.

Cayenne is especially healing to the mucous membrane of the throat and entire alimentary canal. It is specific in sore throat, diphtheria, influenza, and colds. It may be taken in capsules every 2 hours, with food or drink.

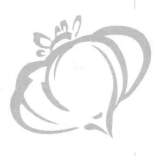

Garlic

Of all the home natural remedies, garlic has been used for the broadest number of diseases and disorders, and no doubt with the greatest success. It has no side effects. Garlic is no doubt the greatest antibiotic or bacteriostatic. It destroys no blood cells; it inhibits the growth of the tumor cells.

In chronic disorders, garlic is useful in high blood pressure, kidney obstructions, hardening of the arteries, senility caused by alkaline toxins, accumulation of cholesterol, hepatitis, inflammation of the bladder, wounds, worms, ulcers, asthma, gastric and intestinal catarrh, sinusitis, etc.

Garlic is a digestive stimulant, an intestinal antiseptic, and a glandular regulator. It is a good source of iodine and thus is beneficial for hypothyroid.

Onions

Onions have the same antibiotic effect as garlic but are not so strong. A cough syrup is made from onions as follows: Put one pint of chopped onion in one-half cup of honey. Keep the mixture warm by placing it in a hot-water bath for 3 hours, and then strain. Take 1 teaspoon of the mixture, as needed, for cough.

A steamed onion poultice over the chest for pneumonia will produce almost unbelievable results. Onions will not blister the skin when made into poultices, but garlic will.

Epsom Salt and Grapefruit Packs

Epsom salt and grapefruit packs have been used with excellent results for a wide variety of disorders, such as colitis, hay fever, bronchial and lung diseases, sore throat, erysipelas, neuritis, mumps, bruises, cuts, abscesses, boils and carbuncles, and blood poisoning.

How to Make and Apply Grapefruit and Epsom Salt Packs:
Grind a whole grapefruit or cut it fine. Add it to 1 to 1 1/2 pints of water, and boil slowly for 15 minutes. Strain. Add all the Epsom salt; the water will dissolve. Wet cloths in the hot solution and apply locally.

Dental Shock and Weakness

It has been noticed that as little as 500 mg of vitamin C given orally prevents shock and weakness after dental extractions.

Eight or ten chlorophyll pearls taken before and after dental extraction will prevent all soreness, shock, and pain, and the gums heal quickly.

Hot Flashes

A daily enema and herbal laxative to cleanse the bowel, and kelp tablets daily, will relieve hot flashes.

Menstruation—Painful

Toxins absorbed into the tissues of the cervix and uterus from the rectum cause inflammation and painful menstruation. Detoxification and rebuilding are indicated. The following herbs are helpful: blue cohosh, black cohosh, and squaw vine.

Warts—To Remove

A wart is a localized benign (nonmalignant) hypertrophy of the skin.

Common warts usually are easy to remove by application of a piece of cotton saturated with castor oil or vitamin E. The saturated cotton is held in place with an adhesive bandage during the night. If possible, keep the bandage on during the day. The wart usually falls off after a few days.

Some warts will not budge with this local application. If not, use asparagus, which contains vitamin B17; it is of the grass family. Four tablespoons of asparagus eaten daily for 2 months usually removes warts; the bandage may also be used. Cereal grasses contain B17, and crude black molasses is also from the grass family.

Stings—Insects

The pain of ant, wasp, yellow jacket, and hornet stings may be relieved by applying vitamin C mixed in honey, after removing the stinger. If you have nothing else, you can mix some dirt or clay with water and apply the mud to the sting. The pain will soon be gone.

Arteriosclerosis (hardening of the arteries)

Dandelion, spinach, and beet tops have been used for hardening of the arteries.

Kidney Stones

Beet tops and beet roots have a dissolving effect on kidney stones. They may be purchased in tablet form.

Sore Throat

Sore throat or acute tonsillitis may be from epidemic streptococcus, from diphtheria infection attended by false membrane in the throat, or streptococcus from milk, spotted sore throat, ulcerated sore throat, or gangrenous pharyngitis.

Acute infectious tonsillitis may be relieved with fomentations (treatment of warm, moist applications, which are better if alternated with cold, and the cold applied for only a minute). Massaging of the throat with lubricants such as Vicks Vaporub or Mentholatum is helpful, with fingers rotating, moving the skin on the deeper tissues. Friction, where the fingers rub over the skin, may irritate.

Massive doses of vitamin C and 5 to 10 garlic pearls every hour will arrest the infection. Lemon juice with cayenne and honey, taken orally, will heal.

Antiphlogistine and cayenne poultices applied at night, covered with woolen cloth, will help to heal through better circulation. Bentonite taken orally every hour will help in any infectious disease.

Arthritis

Alfalfa seed tea, made by simmering a tablespoon of seed in a quart of water, is specific for arthritis. Alfalfa contains over 50 nutrients, and the seed is more potent than the leaves.

Bladder, Kidney, and Ureter Inflammation

Peach leaf tea will eliminate pain and discomfort and heal the entire urinary tract. Dandelion root tea increases the flow of urine and activates the liver.

Peach Leaf Tea:

Into a quart of water, stir about 4 teaspoons of dry peach leaves that have been somewhat crushed. Cover and simmer for 10 to15 minutes; strain and drink a cup four times daily. Garlic may be simmered with the leaves.

Bone Fractures

Lemons have the vitamin C and calcium needed for mending bones. Comfrey is also noted for bone mending.

Honey for Burns

Scars from burns become almost invisible when treated with honey. Vitamin E may be added to the honey.

Antiphlogistine for Burns

Antiphlogistine is a paste made of clay; when applied to burns, it exudes the air and stops the pain immediately, and if applied in time, it will prevent blistering. The burned area should be immersed in cold water until the dressing is applied. This prevents blistering.

Healthy Living, A Holistic Guide

Alum for Burns

Dr. Edwin Wisdom tells us that alum powder, made into a paste with honey or water, will act as an antiseptic in burns.

Oil of Peppermint or Natural Oil of Wintergreen for Burns

Peppermint or Natural Oil of Wintergreen, applied straight or in honey, will relieve the pain of burns immediately. Either of these can be added to any dressing that will stay on.

Acne

Acne may be caused by a deficiency of vitamin B_{12} and folic acid. These nutrients are found in molasses and food yeast. Twelve tablets of high-potency food yeast daily will supply these nutrients in abundance.

Honey applied to acne should help, because it draws pus from boils and carbuncles rapidly. Garlic oil may be added to honey at bedtime.

Vitamin F (Essential Fatty Acids) is necessary for all healthy internal and external tissue. It is found in lecithin.

Bentonite applied to acne is very effective.

Fats, white sugar and white flour products, chocolate, soft drinks, coffee, tea, and tobacco should not be included in the diet.

Vegetables and vegetable juices and broths, fruits, and fruit juices are cleansing, alkaline, nonmucus-forming foods.

Injurious Effects of Tea

Tannic acid is a powerful astringent. It suppresses the digestive juices and causes indigestion. It precipitates pepsin. Dr. Roberts found that tea destroys the action of saliva, and prevents digestion of carbohydrates in the stomach.

Injurious Effects of Coffee

Dr. Edward Smith demonstrated that "Caffeine increases the ability to work, but an increase in fatigue follows. The effect is exhaustion of the cells."

Dr. H.H. Rugby said; "Caffeine is a genuine poison. It tends to be habit forming. It causes permanent disease of the heart in its structural function, and of the nervous system also."

Caffeine tends to raise blood pressure. Dr. Kellogg of Battle Creek Sanitarium observed that the misuse of coffee would raise abnormal blood pressure twenty to forty points.

Tibbles found that coffee cripples the liver. It destroys the glycogenic function of the liver.

17 We Care Health Center
Since 1986

WE CARE Vision and Mission Statement:

We are a Holistic Health Spa and Retreat, providing unique programs designed for personal transformation, enhancing body, mind, and spirit, in a serene desert oasis.

Our experienced team is dedicated to:

- The highest qualilty of service and products
- Integrity, excellence, and compassion
- A comfortable and safe environment, combining ancient and modern techniques
- Inspiring, continued well-being through education and practice

We Care is a fasting and revitalizing retreat that teaches you how to apply all the principles in this book for a healthful lifestyle. The vision of We Care founder Susana Lombardi has grown from humble beginnings into a nationally respected holistic health retreat with an international following that includes Hollywood celebrities, health-conscious North Americans, and medical diplomats from abroad.

We Care is the only facility of its kind with over 5,000 satisfied customers and a 15-year history. Renewing you to a level of health you thought was lost forever is our primary goal. A healing environment makes your stay comfortable and fulfilling.

Unique in all the world, the core processes of the We Care program facilitate proper fasting/cleansing, toxic waste removal, stress release, emotional renewal, and exercise to restore and replenish completely your total well-being.

A complement of nutrition and lifestyle improvement lectures teach how the integration of holistic modalities can create vibrant and lasting fitness from the core being out. As a forerunner in the health movement, Susana teaches little-known, highly effective techniques of self care.

A week at We Care will nurture and transform the whole you. Learning how your body functions best is one of the bonuses of a two-week stay. Make huge strides toward meeting your health goals. Come to We Care soon.

We Care Fasting Retreat in California
- All natural, liquid fasting
- Yoga
- Complete spa facility
- Colonics
- Massages
- Meditation
- Mind-body workshops
- Nutrition classes
- Cooking demonstrations
- Daily juicing
- Energy work
- Guest Speakers
- Rolfing
- Limited accommodations
- Complete home support system

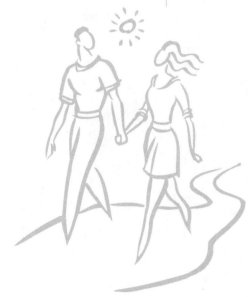

Call 1-800-888-2523 for a FREE catalogue and brochure.

Testimonials

Dear Holistic Colleague:

If you are like most of us, you're working hard promoting wellness on your patients, but having little time to practice what you preach.

I certainly was tired, worn out, a little overweight, and irritable last year when I finally decided to follow the dictum "Physician Heal Thyself." I came to a quiet retreat outside Palm Springs, California for a week of daily massage, juice fasting, colonics, herbs, and gentle exercising. Much to my surprise, I was rejuvenated that week, I lost eight pounds and had done more praying and meditation than I'd been able to do in months at home. My aches and pains disappeared, my brain sharpened, my belly flattened, my body limbered up, and my skin toned wonderfully, all for less than $1,000.00!

Since then I've sent many patients to that spa, people with arthritis, hypertension, digestive problems, and other chronic "TOXIC" conditions. They returned pain-free, drug-free, toxin-free, etc., and on their way to healing. Their improvement is miraculous and lasting, because their life style changes. They were taught vegetarianism and how to lead a healthy life style.

I'm not in any way financially involved in this place, nor am I getting paid for spreading the word. I'm doing this merely to share my wonderful experience with other healers like yourself, so that you and your patients may benefit as we have.

The We Care Center is a family-owned and operated little oasis. A large home, with a pool and great view. It's quiet, isolated, peaceful. The facility has only eleven rooms. It's very, very reasonably priced. And the benefits are well worth any cost. Please take a minute to look at the enclosed material. I truly hope that you avail yourself of this amazingly restoring place. You owe it to yourself and your patients.

Fraternally yours,
Gilbert Manso, M.D.
The Whole Health Center

> *"My aches and pains disappeared, my brain sharpened."*

Dear Susana,

I want to drop you a line and thank you for my incredible week at We Care. My stay with you proved to be exactly what I needed, providing the springboard to completely turn my life around. In addition to cleansing my system, letting go of caffeine, meat, and a host of other wrong habits, I lost twelve pounds, and feel better than I have in ten years! The principles of good nutrition that you live and teach are so simple and sensible, yet are so easy to ignore in our day-to-day lifestyle. My week with you enabled me to experience the benefits of a clean revitalized system and motivated me to maintain my new found "wealth of health" for the rest of my life. I am grateful to you, Manuel, and Bobbe for this gift.

My patients and friends have been commenting on how good I look since I've returned. My skin is clear and vibrant, my eyes are clear, and my energy level is way up. I feel as if I've been given a new lease on life. Also, cleaning out physically seems to have cleared a channel to my heart allowing me better access to my divine nature. The light is emanating from within me much brighter . . . I can feel it and so can others. It's been wonderful!

Thanks again for all your love and inspiration.

In the light,
Steven Heller, D.C.
Clinical Director

> "I feel as if I've been given a new lease on life."

Dear Susana:

I would like to thank you and Manuel for the incredible week that I spent at your place. I am feeling better than I had been for a long time. I feel though that the most important part of the program was all the information that you exposed me to.

To possess and maintain excellent health requires many components and you provide the beginning and the information for a person to accomplish this.

Again many thanks.
Rob
Carlson Travel Group, Inc.

P.S. I will definitely be returning to see you again.

Dear Susana:

I wish to thank you for the courtesy shown me as a travel agent. And also to say a big thank you for all that I learned on my week's stay at We Care Health Center. I have searched for many years and have tried many programs for my health concerns. Your program is the first to give me the tools with which I can help myself with your guidance. Your professionalism and caring manner towards your guests and that of your staff made my visit enjoyable as well as educational. I will have no problem in recommending your Health Center to my clients who are looking for a simple but very effective program for their continued

> "A simple but very effective program."

health care. I am feeling better and I intend to continue following your suggestions, keeping you posted on my progress.

Kindest regards,
Becky Rae
Ask Mr. Foster Travel Service, San Mateo, California 94402

Dear Susana:

I learned even more this time (my second time). Your program is even better and more complete. I feel more revitalized, feel better, look slimmer, and lost twelve pounds.

I live it and will continue better eating habits and will return in six months for a tune-up. Also your video and cassettes are very informative and beneficial! Most of all I want to thank Susana for a wonderful program that really works. I enjoyed my stay here for seven days and learned so much!

All the very best to you,
Bob Bondurant
Sears Point Raceway, Sonoma, CA

Dear Susana:

I truly experienced great gains on your program! I was initially apprehensive about feeling hungry during the week, but that was not the case. I didn't feel hungry all week. Your program is easy to follow—and it works!! I would highly recommend it to anyone who wants an invigorating, rejuvenating retreat from the everyday stress of the world out there.

Sincerely,
Jeff Prager, DDS

Dear Susana:

Thanks for your kind words and for your update on the celebration at your Center. The world is in great need of the healing services you render so professionally and lovingly. You always have my support and best wishes.

Kindest regards,
Michael Klaper, M.D.
Pompano Beach, Florida

"Thanks Susana for a wonderful program that really works."

"Your program is easy to follow—and it works!"

"The world is in great need of the healing services you render."

Recipe Index

Almond Cream, 92
Anchovy Pasta, 77–78
Antipasto Salad, 65
Apricot Pie, 93
Asparagus Soup, 71–72
Avocado, Green Dressing, 58
    Salad, 62

Baked Apples and Pears, 90
Barbecued Peaches with Cream, 92
Basil-Pesto Pasta, 77
Bean Soup, 72
Beans-Vegetable Salad, 66
Beets, Cooked Salad, 67
    with Cloves Salad, 63
Bow Ties with Greens and Mushrooms,
    77

Caffé Latte, 56
Carrots, Grated Salad, 63
    Steamed Salad, 63
Celery Salad, 63
Chinese Ginger Sauce, 60
Chop Suey, 82
Cleansing, Chili Sauce, 59
    Mixed-Green Soup, 70
Cold Mixed Cereal, 51
Corn Salad, Fresh, 63
Creamy Eggplant Casserole, 80
Croquettes, 85
Cucumber Salad, 63, 64

Diced Pineapple and Shredded
    Cabbage Salad, 63
Dynamic Herbal Dressing, 59

Eggplant Spread, 83

Falafel Patties, 85
Fruit Drinks and Smoothes, 55
Fruit Salad, 90
    Raggedy Ann, 92

Ginger Salad, 65
Gourmet Cold Salad, 62
Grains, Plain in Cooker, 87
    Whole, 50
Green Nut Juice, 55

Healthful, Green Dressing, 60
    Mayonnaise, 60
    Tomato Sauce, 75–76

Italian Herbal Dressing, 58

Jicama Salad, 63

"Kelp from the Sea" Dressing, 58

Lasagna, 79
Lemon Garlic Dressing, 58
Linguini with Broccoli and Feta, 78

Millet, Stuffed Onions, 84
    Tomato Loaf, 80

Nut Milk, 50–51

Paella, Fast and Tasty, 88
Papaya Noodles, 76
Pasta, 75
    Al Olio, 76
    Deliciosa, 75
    Radish Leaf Delight, 78
    Summer Dream, 78–79
Peanut Butter Apple Sandwiches, 91–92
Potato, Casserole, 87
    Salad, 64

Quick Energy Soup, 71
Quick Hot Cereal, 51
Quinoa Casserole, 84

Rice, Salad, 67
    and Lentil Salad, 63

Salad Florentine, 66
Sesame Crackers, 91
Spaghetti Squash Salad, 64
Special Sauce for Steamed Vegetables,
    59
Spinach Tofu Salad, 68
Split Pea Stew, 81
Sprouts Salad, 63
Summer Green Salad, 62
Sunburgers, 79–80
Sun Seed Paté, 85
Susana's Super Soup, 70
Sweet and Sour Cabbage, 83
Sweet Potato, Baked, 82
    Sticks, 82

Tabouli, 86
    Casserole, 86
Tahini Dressing, 59
Tasty Legumes Recipe, 86
Tofu, and Onions, 75
    Avocado Spread, 74
    Carrot, Raisin, and Walnut Salad, 74
    Cream, 92
    Pita Pizza, 74
    Pita Dessert, 90
    Spread, 74
Tofurella Cheesecake, 91
Tomato Salad, 66

Vegetable, Juices, 54–55
    Loaf, 79
    Noodle Casserole, 83
    Soup, 88

Watercress and Mushrooms Salad, 63
Winter Hearty Soup, 70–71
Winter Salad, 67
Wholly Guacamole, 60

Zucchini, Casserole with Grains, 81
    Salad, 65